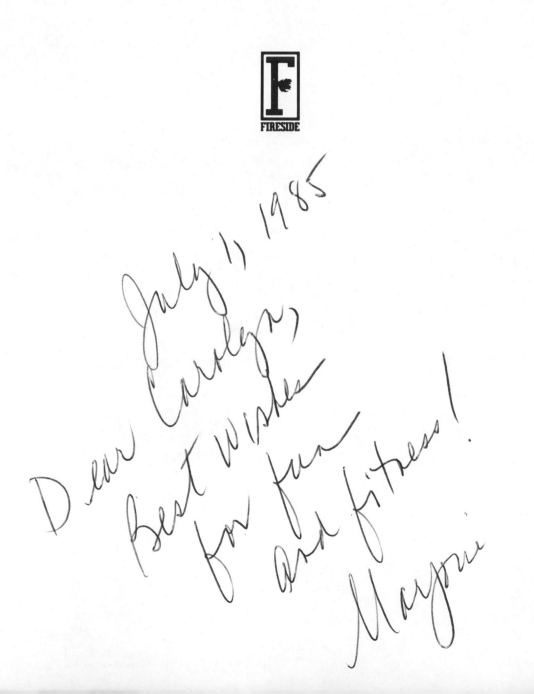

July 1, 1985

Dear Carolyn,

Best wishes
for fun
and fitness!

Margie

GET YOUR BACK IN SHAPE

Marjorie Jaffe
and
Stephanie Cooper

Photography by Susan Daboll

A FIRESIDE BOOK
Published by Simon & Schuster, Inc.
New York

A Fireside Book
Published by Simon & Schuster, Inc.
Simon & Schuster Building
Rockefeller Center
1230 Avenue of the Americas
New York, New York 10020
FIRESIDE and colophon are registered trademarks of Simon & Schuster, Inc.
Designed by H. Roberts Design
Manufactured in the United States of America
Printed and bound by Halliday Lithograph
1 2 3 4 5 6 7 8 9 10

Jaffe, Marjorie.
   Get your back in shape.

   ''A Fireside book.''
   1. Backache—Treatment. 2. Exercise therapy.
3. Physical fitness. I. Cooper, Stephanie. II. Title.
RD768.J34   1984   617'.56   84-1368
ISBN: 0-671-50388-X

Exercise can be stressful and must be performed in the exact manner prescribed in this book. Readers with any medical problems or doubts as to their fitness should only undertake these exercises after consultation with their physician. The authors and the publisher will have no liability, personal or otherwise, for any consequences resulting from the procedures in this book.

Acknowledgments

With heartfelt thanks for loving and sharing, for teaching and inspiration, for patience and support...

Our children—Ian, Bryce and Josh
Our partners—Jerry and Michael
Our parents—Sidney and Rena; Eli and Dvora Cooper
Jacques d'Amboise, Dr. Sonya Weber, Judith Gleason
Our agent—Susan Zeckendorf
Our lawyer and friend—Steven Rand
Our editor—Kathi Paton
Laurie'l and Susan Daboll, who helped to make the book beautiful
The entire Back in Shape Community!

To our growth and realization;
to the curiosity and buoyant spirit that light up our lives.

Foreword

I am delighted with Marjorie Jaffe's clear and direct book of exercises for back care and fitness. I am particularly glad that she is continuing the spirit and content of the work which I began, and which we continued together.

Her quick aptitude for testing, diagnosis and advice has gained her sure, broad experience, which I now see incorporated in this book. I know it will be very useful for people who need exercises to correct back problems and for the general public as well.

This book reflects her considerable work with individual back problems and with testing for muscle weaknesses. She is especially aware of how much harm, injury and discomfort can be caused when people exercise without understanding how their muscles are functioning. I am, therefore, very glad to see the information contained here about proper balance between opposing muscle groups.

Dr. Sonya Weber
Co-inventor of the Kraus-
Weber Physical Fitness Tests

Introduction

How wonderful it is to see the boom in athletic activity that has in these last few years spread so impressively throughout the States. Where once the solitary runner was looked at with apprehension or amusement, now droves of joggers clog the parks and our TV screens are covered with a plethora of bouncing perspiring figures—all energetically calling out the various exercises while smiling furiously. Exercise books and tapes are breaking all records for sales.

All this is affecting and transforming our society. It's amazing when one can remember the days when President Kennedy tried to get the youth of the nation just to try walking more, and failed. Hurray, I say, for I am in favor of a life of physical activity for all.

But—how? and how much? Excess is never good, in exercise as in anything. The orthopedists, chiropractors, podiatrists and osteopaths are reaping the results of athletic excess.

What a delight to find this book espousing a gentle sensible system of exercises aimed at that all-important and most traumatized site, the back. Mrs. Jaffe's lifetime concern and exploration of exercises and posture have resulted in these basic and calming series of beneficial movements.

Bravo, Mrs. Jaffe! You have helped and graced the lives of those who have met you—and now, through these pages, many thousands more.

Jacques d'Amboise
Principal Dancer
New York City Ballet

Contents

GET YOUR BACK IN SHAPE

Preface

For as long as I can remember, I have always taken great joy in the body in movement, whether in dance or sports. And I believe that the freedom to move gracefully and without pain is central to our happiness and vitality throughout our lives. *Back in Shape* first came into being as my studio, the happy product of my lifelong involvement with movement and fitness. It came, as does this book, from my great desire to help other people free themselves from the burdens and limitations of back and neck pain. It reflects many years of training and work experience, particularly under Dr. Sonya Weber, the back-care pioneer. It was after working with her for over ten years that I set out to realize my dream of a studio of my own.

What an exciting and gratifying time that was! But it was frantic and frazzling too. Preparations to open the studio involved enormous decisions, thousands of details and the typical pile-up of last-minute reversals, such as the complete collapse of the wall on which all the studio mirrors were to be installed. I kept my sense of humor throughout by thinking of how tense this business of relaxation was making me. I persevered.

Arrangements were nearly complete, and I had one weekend left to get materials to the printer to announce my arrival to the world. One vital ingredient was missing, however: I needed a name. A good friend came to my rescue. "What is it you most want to accomplish there?" he asked. "To help people conquer their backaches," I replied, "and prevent any recurrences too." I explained that to achieve a healthy back and to put oneself back into shape the secret was to tone and strengthen ALL the body muscles. "Of course!" he cried, imbued with the spirit of my enterprise. "It's *Back in Shape!*" With a little help from my friend I made my printer's deadline. The fliers went into the mail, the ads hit the newspapers, and ever since my doors opened, I have welcomed growing numbers of the out-of-shape, all of whom are quite surprised and equally delighted with how soon and easily results appear. I have cured the discomforts of so many hundreds of back-pain sufferers, probably into the thousands by now, that I am especially eager to share the secrets of my success with you. Come and get your *Back in Shape*. May you banish your back pain, smooth out the tension from your neck, and achieve the strength and fitness you've always wanted!

Marjorie Jaffe

I

Attitudes

No matter what your present state, you were born graceful. You came into the world without a backache, neck pain, stooping shoulders and sagging stomach muscles. But today when you walk down the street, sit at your desk, cook a meal or even take an exercise class—today you may have forgotten that innate natural grace. You may have covered it up with slack muscles here, tension there, with posture that makes you look more like a sagging question mark than the straight strong exclamation point you should stand up and resemble!

Why? Even without life's stress, gravity might be stress enough. A still more important reason is the human tendency to lose awareness of one's physical and mental being. As a result, you slump, you slouch, you hunch, you say good-bye to your inborn capacity to feel fit, energetic and attractive. How shall we change that? Let's take the intelligence that you exercise in every aspect of your life and use it to make your body the best it's ever been—to get you back into the shape you were never in but always knew you could achieve. The secret is a series of slow, thorough exercises. Exercises that will give you pleasure and lasting results because you carry them over into all the movements of your daily life. Exercises that you will UNDERSTAND. Small exercises that you can do in any studio apartment, even in a couchette between Paris and Rome. Indoor exercises. You can, of course, move them out to the lawn if you like.

In order to begin you need to know how your muscles work and how your body ought to be aligned, how the parts rest on one another top to bottom. Understanding is the essential ingredient. An intelligent person resents and resists doing what she or he doesn't comprehend. In order to carry the benefits of specific exercises over to the unconscious movements of everyday life (farewell forever to slouching!) you need to combine movement with consciousness of where your muscles are and how they feel and function. Knowledge added to body alignment is sure to produce lasting muscle tone. That is what I want to help you to achieve.

It is ironic that people go to exercise classes where they work ferociously hard and then go home or to the office slouching against the bus rail or steering wheel to do three hours of phone calls, shoulders hunched—all that good work undone. I want you to take everything you learn horizontally on your exercise mat and apply it vertically in your life. I will teach you intelligent, supereffective exercises and, through them, body awareness. I will show you how to take care of your muscles, to cure their aches and pains so that you can work from head to toe. Your muscles grow weak from lack of exercise—for instance, from sitting for long uninterrupted periods. Tension (which comes from holding your muscles stiff) also weakens muscles and makes you tired. I will help you to bring exercise into your life, to master tension; and I'll show you that not all tension is bad.

In the pages that follow I will teach you the difference between unhealthy tension—the automatic involuntary kind you didn't intend to have—and good, active tension—the kind that gets things done, the positive energy which holds a muscle in the right place and works for you, as in a permanently tighter stomach. Balance is the key word. My aim is to convince you of the pleasure and benefit of balance in your life: a *little* tension along with relaxation to give you comfort and strength. Stress in our everyday lives shortens and weakens our muscles. Yet we want some stress because it keeps excitement up. So we have to have strong muscles to feel fit and healthy and to enjoy our lives and ourselves fully.

Muscle balance means that one muscle never works alone. As in any good relationship, there must be two healthy working parts. With every contraction we need a relaxation. As one muscle tightens, another lengthens. When you see the principles behind the movements in this book, you will begin to apply them to all the movements in your life. You will shape and tone your body in exercise practice, and you'll find yourself doing it almost unconsciously as you stand on a street corner too. You will alter your body movements permanently for the better. You will line up your bones correctly and use your muscles to keep those bones in place. And you'll cure your aches and pains and be healthier for the rest of your life as well.

I am offering you total-body exercises, not isolated parts, because your whole body works together. You'll find the exercises organized into graded levels. The grading is partly based on knowledge and strength, and partly also on sensation. How you are feeling will help you to decide what level best fits your general condition or the particular day. If your sciatic nerve is acting up, go back to Level 1. If you aren't in the mood to exercise, neither are your neuromuscular pathways. But don't cut exercise out altogether—do five sit-ups instead of ten; try Level 1 instead of Level 2, or 2 instead of 3.

Music goes well with exercise: it adds to the aesthetic, graceful side of the experience, to our ability to make our movements pretty. At my studio we always have music in the background. A drill sergeant putting you through sixty leg lifts won't do as much for you as your own knowledge of what you are accomplishing applied to ten. So set the stage with a mood that makes you feel attractive and productive, relaxed and ready to focus on what you're about to do. One of my most satisfying teaching moments came at the end of a class when a student walked over to me, glowing, and said, "I feel so beautiful." Exercise should give you control over your shape and your movements. When you're done with a workout, you should feel taller and more elegant.

Once you're organized and understand your muscles and your body structure in this new and clearer way, I want you to focus on your best, not your worst parts. It's the best that people see in you, particularly if your own attitude is positive. It won't take you long to master the Back in Shape scheme and see positive results. My students report really significant body changes in two to three weeks. I will begin with basic information about your body structure and organization. I've included suggestions about pain and how to eliminate it and some thoughts on how to integrate exercise into a healthy lifestyle. If you are pain-free (and *only* if you are pain-free), you should start with the Organize Yourself section to learn the fundamentals. From there on this book progresses through three increasingly difficult levels of exercise.

Your first step is to see, feel and understand alignment clearly. I'll include only those muscles that you can see, touch and feel easily on your own body. You know, your muscles strengthen your spine and hold your body erect, free to make its movements no matter what your age. Tall or short, thin or heavy, young or old, you need those muscles to move you through your life. My exercises will free you no matter what your age or size. What you strengthen now will keep you freer in the future. Come with me and find new strength and ease. I wish you a happy and successful voyage through the exercises in this book and a future of standing taller and firmer, more comfortably and with much greater pleasure in your total physical being!

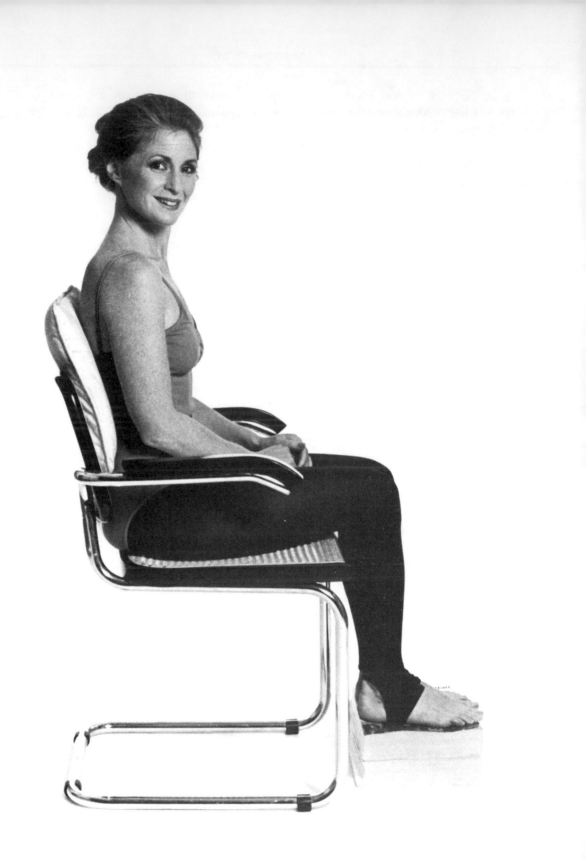

II

Exercise to Live
and
Live to Exercise

In the next chapters you'll see from photos, illustrations and detailed descriptions just how the *Back in Shape* program works. But I couldn't let you go on without a few words on what is probably the most important subject of all—how the exercises fit into your whole life. After all, your exercises take one-half hour of your day at most. What about the remaining twenty-three-and-a-half hours? If you hunch and slump through all that time, your good work will easily be undone. For example, two or three minutes of perfect neck stretches and rotation on your exercise mat cannot possibly make up for three hours spent in conversation with the telephone cradled between your ear and shoulder.

Hunching, slumping and slouching are no better outside the exercise studio than in. In fact, they're worse, because during exercise you're *aware* of your body. Away from exercise, perhaps you've always tuned out and lost consciousness of how your body is aligned. There's no need to do that any longer. In fact, my very point is that you *must* TAKE YOUR CHECKPOINTS WITH YOU TO THE REST OF YOUR LIFE. Good alignment should become as much your habit as how you brew the morning coffee.

You will learn that along with alignment the most valuable body habit you can develop is relaxation. Here are some hints for including its benefits in your nights and days: Most of us spend huge amounts of time sitting down. Slumping when you sit makes the back muscles compress and irritates the nerves. To ease the strain of sitting, place a phone book in front of your chair under your feet—one book if you're from New York City, and several if you're from a smaller town. This will raise your knees to a level higher than your hips and thus relax stiff lower-back muscles.

Another hint is to place a pillow in the space between your upper back and the back of your chair. Make sure your buttocks go all the way to the back. This way you won't slump, and your checkpoints will be in line. You'll actually feel lighter—almost a floating sensation. You'll be so comfortable in this position that you may *want* to take a job that requires sitting. However, sitting or standing, don't ever stay in one position for too long. Hours in the car, for instance, can be very wearing unless you make occasional stops to stretch and loosen up.

Sometimes back pain may result from your legs being of uneven lengths. We're not all symmetrical, although for comfort and muscular good health we should be. The longer leg causes a higher hip on that side, and makes the spine curve sideways when it should be straight. In this state sitting can be uncomfortable. To correct the problem put a thin paperback book under the lower hip to straighten the spine. The relief will be remarkable. (The book should be about one-half inch thick.)

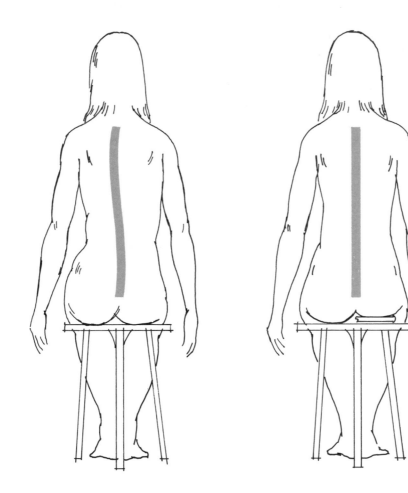

Unevenness can also plague your shoulders. The culprit here is often that heavy shoulder bag you carry, filled to bursting. To keep it from slipping down you hike your shoulder up and thereby produce a permanently higher shoulder. The solution? It's best to wear the strap across your chest. Second best, divide the load.

Welcome relief from back pain may also be found by changing mattresses. If you awaken stiff and sore each morning, it may be that your bed is either too hard or too soft. Softness, which is bad because it gives you no support, is easy to cure with a quarter-inch beaverboard or plywood sheet placed between the mattress and box spring. On the other hand, if the surface is too hard, it's equally harmful because it doesn't allow your muscles to relax. My advice here is to take a trip to the bedding store, kick off your shoes and your self-consciousness, and give all the mattresses a thorough testing. Don't look for spartan hardness, but make sure to choose support with plenty of cushioning.

Now that I've put exercise into the total context of your life, now that I've discussed sitting and lying down in comfort, it's time to move on to the good work that will cure your pain and increase your tone and fitness. Remember, you must take what you are about to learn into the larger sphere of your whole life.

III

Organize Yourself

How's your posture? Chances are, your mother made "Stand up straight!" a constant growing-up refrain. Mom was right. The benefits of standing straight are well known: balanced muscles make us feel tall and trim, pretty and well-put-together. And what's right aesthetically turns out to be right therapeutically too. With muscles holding our bones in good position there's room for the healthy functioning of our internal organs; our nerves don't get pinched and irritated, and aches and pains are few.

It sounds so simple—"Stand up straight." And it *is* simple *if* we are aware of the basic ingredients that create body alignment. Once you can isolate (both intellectually and by sensation) the body regions that control alignment, once you are easily aware of how those regions hang together, then you'll be in charge of your posture in a relaxed and natural way. You'll find yourself constantly and casually straightening and relaxing cramped muscles as part of your spontaneous body movement. Keeping correct alignment is a process similar to driving a car. Gusts of wind push a car out of its straight path down the highway, just as physical and mental stresses push our bodies out of line. As drivers we steer almost unconsciously, knowing by feel how to keep in our lane. In this chapter I will show you how to keep your body in line in much the same way.

After all, life offers us much harder tasks than standing. Some of you ski or skate or play tennis; most of you swim. A number may still know how to waltz or tango. Obviously you've already accomplished feats way beyond that first great human achievement—standing up. It's the one that separates us from most of the animal kingdom. And being so basic and assumed a stance, it is the one we need to remind ourselves about, the one to perfect because all movements flow from it. There are five basic body regions that provide the components of proper alignment. If you organize yourself from the bottom up, you'll stand correctly, which is essential if any exercise is to be effective. Let's try. The following steps correspond to the numbers on the diagram. Stand sideways to the mirror:

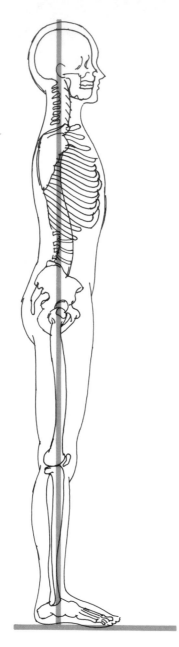

1. Place Weight Forward Toward Balls of Feet.

The center of your body (your center of gravity) should be directly above the arches of your feet. (Note the foot exercises at the end of Level 1. Our feet support us and need special attention.)

2. Make Legs Softly Straight.

Don't clamp your knees into a ramrod-stiff position—that will throw your weight backward and arch your back too much. Make sure your knees are relaxed over your ankles.

3. Line Up Pelvic Girdle Over Knees.

Don't suck in your breath to keep your stomach in—it won't work. As soon as your mind wanders, which undoubtedly will be immediately, out goes the belly. Instead, know that there are three particular sets of muscles that hold your pelvic bones in place. Don't worry about their names. DO touch your belly where the diagrams and explanations indicate:

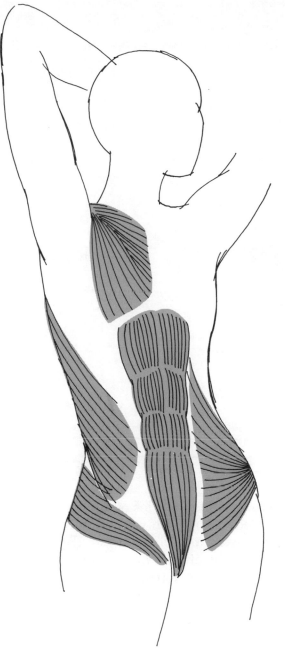

a. *rectus*—ties to the pubic bone and each rib. Feel a broad rectangular muscle running up and down from the ribs to the pubic bone along the front of your body. When this muscle is firm, your stomach doesn't sag. Draw your ribs together and feel the hard muscle between them.

b. *oblique*—diagonal muscle bands that crisscross at the navel. Two attach from the ribs to the navel, and the other two go from the hips to the belly. Put your hands on your belly where the diagram indicates the muscles. Draw your ribs together and feel them harden.

c. *transverse*—a two-inch band across the waist. Poke with a finger to find this stiff band of muscle. Don't worry if it's soft. The exercises will develop it in very little time.

Because we're not four-footed, we need these muscles for support. When they are taut and strong, they take all the pressure off the back, which no longer has to do their job for them. Draw those muscles in. Hold them (don't forget to breathe). Backache, bye-bye!

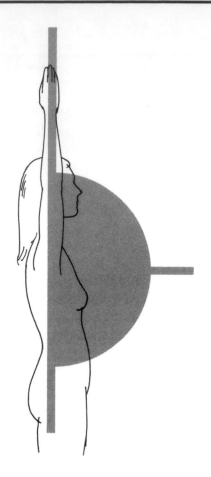

4. Center Rib Cage Directly Over Pelvic Girdle

Lift your arm straight up in a 180-degree angle to find the muscles of your chest. If your angle isn't perfectly straight, you need to lengthen your pectoral muscles. These are the muscles of the thorax, or chest. Run a fingertip up the front of your ribs to your collarbone and continue to the end of the shoulder. The pectoral ties from that point diagonally down like a fan across the chest to each rib. You know you need work on your pectorals if your shoulders are rounded, if you can't close a back zipper easily or reach a book on a high shelf. When the pectoral muscles are stretched and strong, they lift our ribs and keep them erect and straight. Visualize them as a fan of rubber bands spreading across the chest. If the rubber bands are stretched, your shoulders are straight. If your muscles are tight and weak, the rubber bands stay short, and your shoulders are pulled forward. In that case you may even have an (entirely correctable) hump of muscle across the back of your neck.

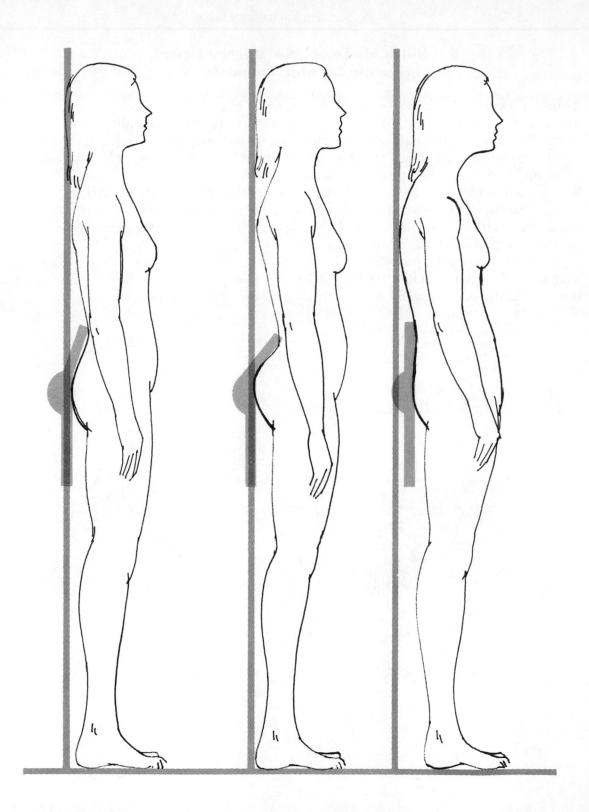

5. Hold Chin Level—Not Up, Not Down. Line Up Ear with Shoulder.

Think of leveling your gaze and looking straight ahead. We are now talking about the cervical, or neck, region. The most important muscle here is the trapezius. It forms the back of the neck and upper shoulders, a classic place for tension to strike you. When the trapezius is stretched and strong, it holds your head up straight above your shoulders and trunk. When tense and weak, it forces your neck to curve forward—not a graceful or comfortable position. Unlike our furry four-footed friends who keep their noses to the ground to sniff, we do best with our heads held high. Straighten your neck; feel a string pulling up the top of your skull as your neck muscles lengthen up the back. Always think of a large, open space stretching up between your shoulder and ear. LET YOUR NECK HOLD YOUR HEAD UP. Notice, please, that your chin should be *down*, and the back of your head in the same line as your upper back.

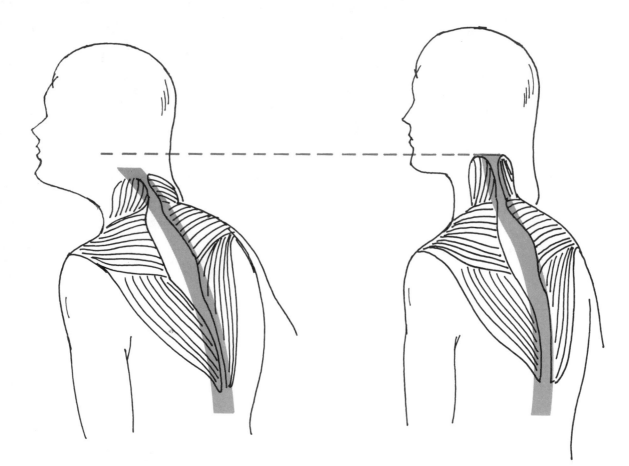

NOW YOU ARE ALIGNED!

As you read through the exercises that follow, you will see constant references to these five regions. They are regions for your mind as well as your body. They are *checkpoints*, a word that will become part of your life. Your checkpoints will help you to visualize your body so that you can build it. In fact, think of yourself as an elegant pile of building blocks, one placed upon another, balanced and straight. Know also that even before you begin, you have muscle tone that is developed, although you may feel quite flabby. Every gesture you make requires the tensing of a muscle or a group of muscles. Try picking up a pencil with limp fingers. It can't be done! We tense our muscles to do tasks. That tension is a healthy, natural way to overcome gravity. When our astronauts have returned to Earth from prolonged periods of weightlessness, they have come back with seriously depleted muscle strength caused by the absence of gravity. There was nothing in Space for their muscles to work against.

Thus the same gravity that weighs us down also helps to hold us up. As our muscles work to counteract its force, they stimulate the bones to produce essential calcium. Please note, therefore, that although our present culture discourages tension, it has its healthy place and use. As you learn to employ tension, you gain in the good feeling of self-mastery and vitality. As you isolate muscles and learn to work them, you will also learn how to let go of their stiffness. The secret of a healthy balance, I repeat, is awareness. Be aware that as we tense one muscle, or contract it, we are simultaneously lengthening another. For example, if you bring your hand to your shoulder, your forearm muscles shorten as your back arm muscles lengthen. Every movement, then, has two parts that create balance. I will teach you balance in the exercises that follow.

I particularly want you to know that exercise does not have to hurt to be good. Quite the opposite. Pain is a signal from your nerves to your brain that what you are doing is wrong for you. It is vital for you to distinguish the feeling of exertion from the feeling of pain. It is fine to push yourself on to higher and higher levels of accomplishment. But it is *always* essential to respect nature's signals so that you avoid injury.

Perhaps most important to discuss before we begin the work of specific exercises is the issue of quality versus quantity. A person can do fifty sit-ups and finish, gasping for air, sweaty, *feeling* thoroughly exercised. But if that person did the sit-ups improperly by just throwing his or her arms forward, there wasn't one good productive movement in the lot. Most if not all the work was probably accomplished by the poor old aching back. A sit-up has value if your stomach muscles do the job. No matter what the exercise, if you know *what* you're trying to accomplish, you can concentrate on the muscle you need and make *it* do its proper job. (Then watch how fast the waistlines on your clothes grow looser!) Now look again at the diagrams of the muscles and of the aligned body and its five regions. Organize your body again so you know its parts. Find them by touch and awareness.

Let's also investigate your muscle tone a bit. I don't suggest you try to test stomach strength through exercise—if your stomach muscles are weak, you may strain your back. Instead, poke around a little with your finger. When a muscle has good tone, it feels resilient to the touch. Your fingertip should bounce off, not sink in. For instance, the transverse muscle should feel like a diagonal cord at your waist between your lowest rib and your hip. If you pull in your waist, rather than suck in your breath to button your skirt, you should feel your transverse. Look down—if your waist is flabby, it looks flabby. Strong muscles look strong.

Muscle tests (such as the Kraus-Weber Tests developed at Columbia Presbyterian Medical Center by my teacher, Dr. Sonya Weber) have revealed that most people have weaker front than back muscles. And weak abdominals are the major cause of backaches. You will find that the exercises that follow are designed to strengthen your abdominal muscles while at the same time lengthening and relaxing those of the back. (Balance again!) The Level 1 exercises which you are about to learn are geared to the minimum fitness you need. They are also a vital introduction to my method, developed out of years of teaching and culled from the best of many highly respected approaches to exercise and fitness. These exercises really work. You will strengthen yourself on all levels, but the first is the most basic. It is the point at which to begin unless you are in pain (in which case, consult the pain section that follows). And it is the place to which you should return on days when you're not feeling your best, even though you may have mastered Levels 2 and 3.

As you proceed through the exercises, watch your body and touch it. Feel the parts work. Check with your hands that your pelvis is straight, that your ribs are directly over it, that your neck is straight along its back, that a nice, large space is open between your ear and shoulder. And notice, too, the importance of breathing in exercise. Sending oxygen-rich blood to your muscles makes their movements flow and increases your relaxation. I'll give you breathing directions as we go along.

Now—put on shorts, a sweatsuit or a leotard, whatever is most comfortable. You need a firm surface to lie on, but one with some give. So roll out a towel on the rug, use an exercise mat, or put your quilt down on the wooden floor. Turn on the music, adjust the lights, line yourself up (organize yourself), and here we go!

IV

Before You Begin,
Be Comfortable

The most important rule to follow for exercise is to BE COMFORTABLE. Pain is a message from your brain to your body that something is wrong. Therefore, before we begin the work of stretching and strengthening, it is essential for you to understand when that work can safely be done. There is no doubt that any movement you make which causes you pain is not safe for you and should not be done. So the first ingredient for successful exercise is *awareness* of your body—pay attention to it, listen to it, learn about it, and it will tell you what your safe limits are. By rushing into exercise, by galloping through complicated sequences you don't understand, you're sure to injure yourself. By taking things one step at a time you'll get to know your body better—its weaknesses and strengths (I'm quite sure you have *both*), and ultimately your progress will be quicker and more complete.

If at this very moment you've got an achy spot—particularly in your neck and shoulders or your lower back—DON'T go ahcad to Level 1. Please use the following suggestions to get yourself ready to begin: First, only do those things that are comfortable. (This is as true in exercise as it is in life, especially with regard to heavy lifting.) DON'T LIFT! Call someone strapping—your spouse, your neighbor, your adolescent son or daughter. Know your limits.

If you have a specific discomfort, I recommend any mild anti-inflammatory medicine like aspirin or one of its substitutes because a sore muscle may indicate an inflamed nerve. Of course, any medication you take should have the approval of your doctor. Why do I believe in aspirin and related drugs? Basically because muscle pain is a cyclical phenomenon, and to cure it you must break the cycle. An ache in a muscle usually comes from its being too tense. Because muscles and nerves are closely intertwined in our bodies, a tense muscle will irritate a nerve. The irritated nerve then causes the muscle to tighten even more, in response to pain. And so the cycle prolongs itself and can only be corrected by breaking the chain: reduce the inflammation and discomfort, and the muscle will begin to relax. So don't put off that aspirin, and don't overdo it either.

Another suggestion to help you regain your comfort is to find the most comfortable position possible and try to make it more comfortable. If your lower back is painful, try lying on your side with a pillow between your thighs. This will make your top leg level with your spine and will take pressure off irritated nerves. A second position that is often helpful is on your back with pillows under your knees. Try one, two or even three so that your knees bend and take pressure off the back and its irritated nerves. How many pillows do you need? However many feel good. Later you will notice that these positions are similar to two of our most basic Level 1 exercises—the Side Slide and the Pelvic Tilt, both of which are designed for relaxation and gentle strengthening.

There are no hard-and-fast rules about how to lie. Whatever position gives you a better night's sleep, use it and enjoy it! Generally, I don't recommend sleeping on your stomach because it tends to increase the sway in your back. You'll know if that applies to you because you'll feel it.

You can also help an aching back or neck with moist heat. It penetrates to sore muscles much more effectively than dry heat, to which it is therefore preferable. Hot baths and showers (those shower massage machines have worked wonders for some people) and commercially available moist heating pads are all helpful.

On the other hand, if you are in pain from a muscle spasm or trauma, you might try an ice pack. (Use it according to your doctor's instructions.)

It is wisest and safest if you are uncomfortable to begin your work with the relaxation section of Level 1. You can do the relaxation exercises three times each day while you are in pain. It's only a five-minute program. Take a look at it when you are ready to begin. Notice the Side Slide, which I just mentioned. You can do it with or without your raising your leg. Look at the Relaxation and Organization, and at the Pelvic Tilt. DO WHAT IS COMFORTABLE, and when your pain is gone, go on to the rest of the program.

V

Before, During and Afterthoughts

- Always loosen for as long as you tighten.
  Remember relaxation movements:
    —Wobble head to loosen neck.
    —Shrug shoulders to release tension.
    —Never shake briskly to relax a muscle.
- Your slogan: "With my belly in and my neck straight. . . ."
- Always make a nice, big, open space between your ear and shoulder.
- Breathing: Never let breathing instructions interfere with learning an exercise. (That's why we've put them after the directions to all levels). NEVER HOLD YOUR BREATH. Remember to breathe in and out regularly as you are in the learning phase. Then try to coordinate the breathing with the movements, once you have mastered them fully.
- A healthy back (Position 1) is neither too curved (Position 2) nor too straight (Position 3). This illustration shows the indicated angle of your pelvic tilt—how much you sway in or out—in relation to a straight 180-degree line. Your spinal nerves emerge from the bony processes of each vertebra. If you tilt too much or too little, they can infringe on each other and cause pain.

- A straight back (Position 3) is weaker than a curved back. The straight back causes the center of gravity of the body to be pushed forward. In order to maintain erect posture the straight back must work harder than normal. Thus it is always tense. When tension such as this cannot be released, it leads to irritation.

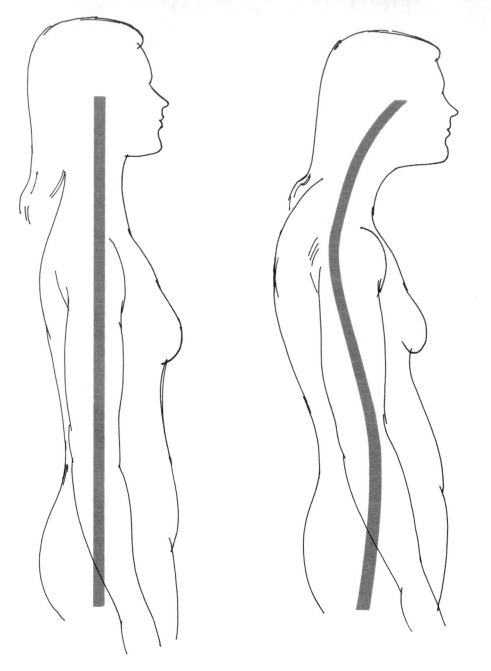

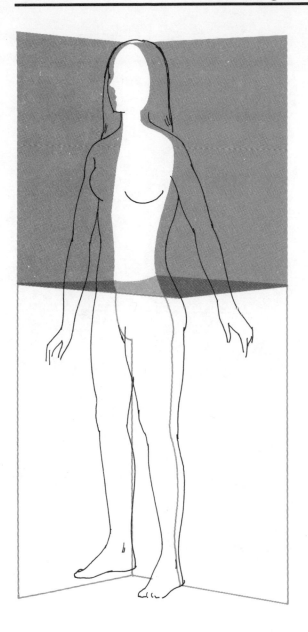

Think of your center: Divide your body into three planes, and picture the point where they intersect. As you pull up to set your posture throughout the exercises, always think of this center spot, and draw up through it.

    —Plane 1—symmetrical right and left halves

    —Plane 2—top and bottom halves

    —Plane 3—front and back halves

It is important not only to think of your outward appearance, but to *concentrate on your inside* as you draw up through the center.

VI

Level 1:
Basic Exercises

When you lie down to exercise, it is easy to achieve the lovely straight look of perfect alignment because you don't have to contend with the stress of gravity. Remember the feeling of straightness in all these positions, and apply it to your standing self. Check your alignment regularly as you work.

Let's begin Level 1 with the alignment steps. Sideways to the mirror,

1. Rock a bit between your toes and heels to find the center of your feet.
2. Keep knees softly straight, not locked.
3. Tummy in—so center of pelvis stands directly over center of feet.
4. Ribs up and straight with center of chest over center of pelvis.
5. Back of neck stretching tall; back of head in line with upper back; make a nice big, open space between your earlobe and shoulder.
6. Drop shoulders and let gravity pull them down.

Check this lovely posture in the mirror. Wait two seconds, and repeat, facing the mirror: This time think of pulling up through the center of your body as if a soda straw were running up and down inside you. As you repeat the alignment steps 1 to 6, think of drawing in on that straw, with all your body fluids flowing in and up.

Now take your alignment with you to the floor, and let's begin.

1. SIDE SLIDE—3X EACH

Purpose

TO ELIMINATE LOWER BACK
PAIN—gentle stretching of back muscles to
take pressure off irritated nerves in lower
back.

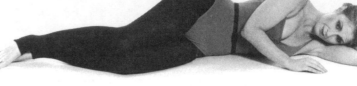

Position

a. Lie comfortably on one side.
b. Gently bend lower leg and rest upper leg
   in space behind knee.
c. Small pillow or lower arm folded under
   head to keep cervical spine straight.
d. Be certain to relax and *let go* of muscles
   in body.

Directions

a. Raise top leg to level of hip.
b. Gently bend knee toward chest, keeping
   at same hip level, and feel back stretch.
c. Slide leg back to starting position—hold
   still and feel weight of leg.
d. Now let leg drop down and *let go*.
   Wobble to loosen body.
e. Repeat (a) through (d) on other side.

Note

Pause between each movement to relax
body. Bend knee toward chest only as high
as is NOT painful. If raising leg to hip level
is painful, *DON'T*! Instead, stretch the leg
while resting it on the bent knee, and do the
Side Slide without lifting.

2. RELAXATION AND ORGANIZATION— 3X EACH

Purpose
TO ELIMINATE BODY TENSION—to make body comfortable for exercise; to put you in touch with the feeling of alignment.

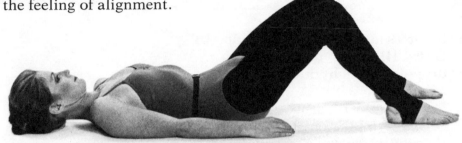

Position
a. Lie on back with knees bent, feet flat on floor, hip-width apart.
b. Small pillow under head if necessary for comfort.
c. Place hands on belly, let it sink in; and have a concave feeling from ribs down to pubic bone.
d. BACK OF NECK STRETCHED OUT LONG (lots of space between ear and shoulder)—line of sight between knees, not up at ceiling.

Directions
Tension is to *hold* a muscle. Relaxation is to *let go*. Let a sense of relaxation wash over you as you complete these movements.
a. Deep breathing—inhale deeply through nose and feel ribs rise. Exhale through mouth and feel ribs lower. Keep inhalation and exhalation time equal. *Let go* and relax before each of the next inhalations. Remember to keep belly in, to move ribs up and down with breathing, and to keep back of neck straight.

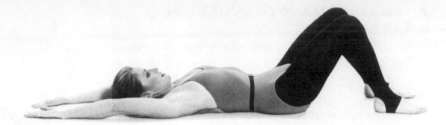

b. Same as (a) with arms stretching UP OVER HEAD on inhalation and dropping straight down one at a time on exhalation.

c. Same as (a) with arms stretching SIDEWAYS up along floor on inhalation, then sideways down on exhalation. Let shoulders and arms wobble on the way down. Keep palms facing toward ceiling as arms sweep up and down.

d. Wobble head lightly, like a feather, to loosen neck muscles; then slowly let head drop to one side and *let go;* then drop head to other side and *let go.*

e. Wobble and shrug shoulders to loosen and relax.

f. Keep heels on floor as you let each leg slide down slowly; slide until you can *let go* and drop leg! Wobble legs and *let go* of muscles.

3. PELVIC TILT—5X SLOWLY

Purpose
TO PREVENT BACK PAIN—to develop a strong, flat stomach and take pressure off lower back; to tighten transverse muscle (waist) and entire set of lower abdominals.

Note

People with straight backs (without a sway or lumbar curve) should do the pelvic tilt ONLY as an isometric to flatten the tummy and tighten the waist (transverse muscle). DO NOT squeeze the buttocks—this only adds to the straightness. Straight backs are weaker than curved backs and need to be strengthened. To do so substitute Leg Extension for Pelvic Tilt on Stomach (after Position 2).

Position 1:   PELVIC TILT ON BACK

   Lie on back, knees bent; feet on floor, hip-width apart.

Directions

a. Begin by tensing inner thighs and groin area.

b. Press in lower belly and tighten waist.

c. Press all tummy muscles in toward belly button; with your hands, feel a *concave tummy*.

d. DO NOT HOLD BREATH!

e. Do not lift buttocks, but squeeze together to "set" this position. (Buttocks will automatically lift slightly, and you will feel a tilting up of the pelvis.)

f. Feel for the "cords" at sides of waist; (transverse muscle) feel an east-side to west-side cut along waist; feel a nicely concave tummy.

g. Hold for a slow count of 5—DO NOT HOLD YOUR BREATH—and then *let go*, pause in between and repeat.

Position 2: PELVIC TILT ON STOMACH

a. Lie on stomach; rest forehead on folded hands.

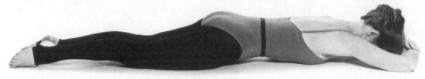

Directions

a. Pinch buttocks together and press down.
b. Pull in transverse and feel tummy lift off floor as back straightens and becomes flat (this is the reverse of the Pelvic Tilt).
c. Keep upper back quiet and DO NOT HOLD BREATH!

Leg Extension

(For people with straight backs, substitute for Pelvic Tilt on Stomach.)

Purpose

TO STRENGTHEN LOWER BACK MUSCLES AND DEVELOP A HEALTHY CURVE.

Note

DO ONLY IF THERE IS *NO* PAIN.

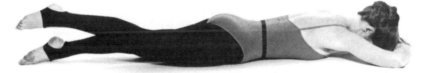

Position

a. Lie on stomach; rest head on folded hands.
b. Keep upper back quiet.

Directions

a. Keeping hip down, slowly raise single leg (only as high as is comfortable).
b. Put down gently and *let go*.
c. Alternate, three times each leg; when stronger, add double leg lifts, alternating three times.

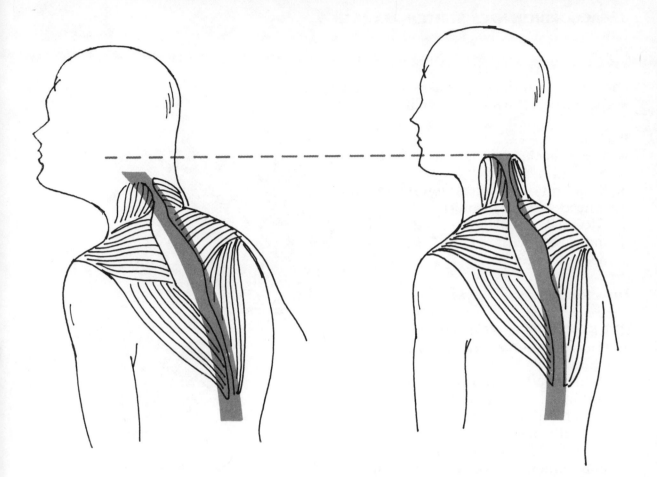

A Note About the Neck

There are seven cervical vertebrae in your neck. It is vital to make this area of your spine (we call it the cervical spine) straight so that the nerves can emerge freely from the vertebrae without being irritated. Remember, muscles move your bones. When neck muscles become too short, they pull the skull back, pressing the bones together and irritating the nerves. As a result—that classic pain in the neck. A long, relaxed neck not only looks graceful, it feels comfortable.

4. ACCORDION NECK STRETCH—3X EACH

Purpose

TO ELIMINATE NECK PAIN—to lengthen and strengthen the trapezius muscle, which keeps the cervical spine straight.

Position

a. Lie on back, knees bent; feet on floor, hip-width apart.
b. Small pillow or folded towel under neck if necessary for comfort.
c. ORGANIZE YOURSELF—start each movement with "My belly in and my neck straight. . . ."

Directions

NECK STRETCH *WITH* HANDS

a. Put hands out in front of you and bend elbows.
b. Hold on to back of head at top.
c. Pull head forward slightly off mat and stretch cervical spine (back of neck).
d. Carefully place down seventh cervical—the bump at top of spine—then, one vertebra at a time, lower until head is flat down, cervical spine as straight as comfortable. (Use pillow under head to "raise floor" until muscle becomes stretched enough to reach floor by itself.)

NECK STRETCH *WITHOUT* HANDS

a. Tummy in, neck straight.
b. Slide back of neck as straight down into floor as possible (chin will go down as head bends forward). DO NOT LIFT! Feel back of neck stretch and elongate. Imagine a sponge underneath neck; imagine pressing sponge down into floor. Press, pause; press, pause. Always wobble to loosen.

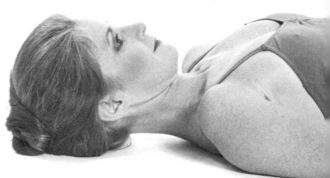

5. KNEE HUG—3X EACH

Purpose
TO RELAX AND STRETCH LOWER BACK
MUSCLES.

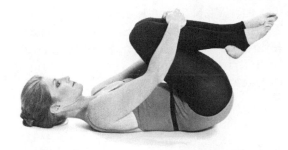

Position
a. Lie on back, knees together and bent on
chest, hands hugging knees
and/or
b. Lie on back, knees open and bottoms of
feet together, hands holding ankles.

Directions
Position a. Hug knees gently with hands,
press toward chest and sway softly.
Position b. Press feet in toward crotch
gently with hands and sway softly.

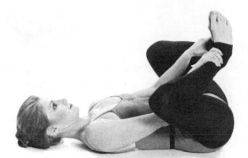

6. KNEE KISS—3X EACH,
ALTERNATING KNEES

Purpose
TO STRETCH HAMSTRING MUSCLES
AND TIGHTEN ABDOMINALS.

Position
a. Lie on back, knees bent; feet on floor.
b. Arms at sides.

Directions
a. Raise head and left knee.
b. Left hand under buttocks to help.
c. Squeeze belly in to help lift ribs.
d. Try to touch forehead to knee.
e. Keeping belly in, slowly lower head and
knee.

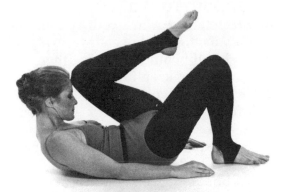

Note
Use upper back and neck muscles to lift
head so neck doesn't tire.

Coordinate Breathing
a. Inhale on way down.
b. Exhale on way up.

7. BASIC HAMSTRING STRETCH— ALTERNATE 3X EACH LEG

Purpose

TO PREVENT BACK PAIN CAUSED BY
TIGHT HAMSTRINGS—to stretch and
lengthen muscles of backs of legs (tight
hamstrings are one of the principal causes
of backache).

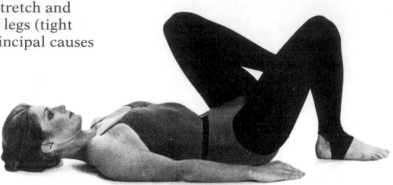

Position

a. Lie on back, knees bent; feet on floor.
b. Work one leg at a time with opposite
knee bent.
c. Belly in (remember concave feeling);
back of neck straight (chin down);
shoulders down.

Directions

a. Bring knee toward chest, but DO NOT
LIFT BUTTOCKS.
b. Stretch leg toward ceiling, foot loose,
only as high as knee stays straight.
c. Feel pull behind knee—neither lock nor
bend knee; keep it softly straight.
d. Gently bounce leg toward you several
times like a screen door gently knocking
in a breeze—then,
e. Bend knee, put foot down, let leg slide
and DROP down.
f. Wobble to loosen and repeat.

8. LEG LIFTS ON SIDE— 3X EACH

Purpose
TO TIGHTEN THE *LOWER* BELLY.

Position
a. Lie on side, body in a completely straight line (CHECKPOINTS: ear, shoulder, hip, knee, ankle).
b. Bend elbow to support head in hand.

Directions
a. Tighten transverse before each leg lift.
b. SLOWLY raise leg straight up and down (with resistance* to increase difficulty) as you
c. Keep knee forward—don't let it turn up toward ceiling; pull up through center of body as you lower leg.
d. Keep hip rotated in—this tightens buttocks.
e. Allow NO sway in body—the tighter you hold your belly, the less you move.
f. Hold weight of leg by tightening lower belly.

Coordinate Breathing
a. Breathe in to begin.
b. Exhale as you slowly stretch leg up.
c. Inhale just after you lower.

*Resistance
a. As you raise, think of heavy weight on top of leg; press against heavy weight.
b. As you lower, think of pressing down against heavy metal bar.
c. Think of magnetic pull between inner thighs, and keep turning leg in.

9A. CURL-BACK—5X EACH

Purpose
TO STRENGTHEN ABDOMINAL
MUSCLES, ESPECIALLY RECTUS
MUSCLE—weak abdominals are THE
principal cause of backache.

Position
a. Begin in sitting position, knees bent; feet
   flat on floor, hip-width apart.
b. Arms loose at sides—the less you use
   your arms, the harder your stomach
   muscles work and the *more effective* the
   exercise.
c. Head bent forward, cervical spine
   stretching.

Directions
a. DO NOT LET FEET LIFT OFF FLOOR.
b. Roll back slowly toward floor (ONLY AS
   LOW AS YOU DO *NOT* FEEL STRAIN)
   and stop before lower back touches floor.

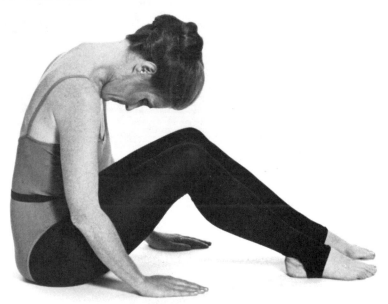

c. Set tummy muscles to hold position.
d. Tense inner thighs and groin area; press down hard in ribs and belly.
e. Keep *letting go* in shoulders and arms.
f. Hold for a slow count of 5, then pull forward to starting position (with equal pull in belly AND inner thighs).
g. Press in groin and lower belly to release lower back before repetition; rock gently.

Coordinate Breathing

a. Exhale as you roll back.
b. Inhale as you pull yourself forward.

Note

The less you use your shoulders to help you, the tighter you'll make your stomach, the more productive this exercise.

REMEMBER: the rectus muscle ties from each rib to the pubic bone—by pulling it in you pull your ribs forward and thus can sit up.

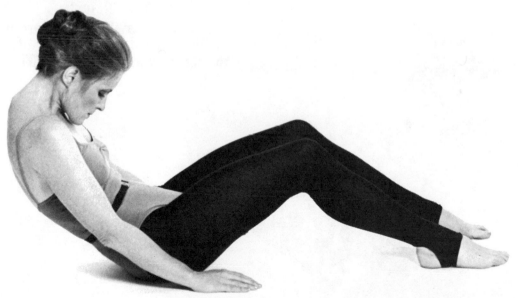

9B. DIAGONAL CURL-BACK—3X EACH SIDE

Purpose
TO STRENGTHEN ABDOMINAL MUSCLES, especially the diagonal obliques (four muscles that crisscross at center of waist).

Position
a. Same as step (a), Curl-Back 9A.
b. Twist upper body to right and look over right shoulder.
c. Bend head down to stretch cervical spine.
d. Drop arms loosely down to right.
e. *NOTE:* when you change sides, repeat position, but move head and arms to left.

Directions
a. DO NOT LET FEET LIFT OFF FLOOR.
b. Roll diagonally back.
c. Keep twisting and set muscles—feel a strong effort in waist.
d. Tense inner thighs and groin area; press down hard in ribs and belly.
e. Keep *letting go* in shoulders and arms.

f. Hold for a slow count of 5, then pull diagonally forward to starting position (with equal pull in belly AND inner thighs).

g. Press in groin and lower belly to release lower back before repetition.

Note

Because this exercise requires enormous effort, it is very important to relax between each Curl-Back: wobble from side to side; feel bones under your bottom; give your back a good forward stretch.

10. REPEAT KNEE HUG (No. 5) AND RELAXATION (No. 2).

11. REPEAT SIDE SLIDE (No. 1) AND RELAXATION (No. 2).

12. SHOULDER CIRCLES— 5X SLOWLY AND CORRECTLY

Purpose

TO ELIMINATE UPPER BACK AND NECK PAIN—to eliminate round shoulders by lengthening pectoral muscles; to tighten muscles that hold shoulder blades and spine (rhomboid muscles).

Note

It's easy to do this exercise completely ineffectually. It can look right, but it won't do you any good unless you feel a specific tightening *between* shoulder blades. BE CERTAIN TO RELAX AND *LET GO* BETWEEN EACH STEP: Try shoulder shrugs, head rolls, deep breathing. (Directions for head rolls follow this exercise.)

Position
a. Sit cross-legged on the floor if comfortable; or sit on a chair.
b. Belly tucked in.
c. Chest in front of stomach—keep weight forward.
d. Back of neck straight; back of head in line with upper back; chin level.
e. Shoulders relaxed and down—nice big open space between ear and shoulder.

Directions
a. Bend arms and place fingertips on shoulders.
b. Slowly make backward circles.

Note
This movement is done by shoulder, *not* elbow; so check that shoulder stays farther *back* than elbow.

    1) Begin with a slight lift.
    2) Keep circling motion behind you.
    3) Slowly roll all the way back.
    4) Feel shoulder blades come together and blend movement to
    5) Pull down, keeping shoulders *back* (the movement is both back and down).
    6) *Let go*, and return to starting position.
    7) PAUSE, and repeat.

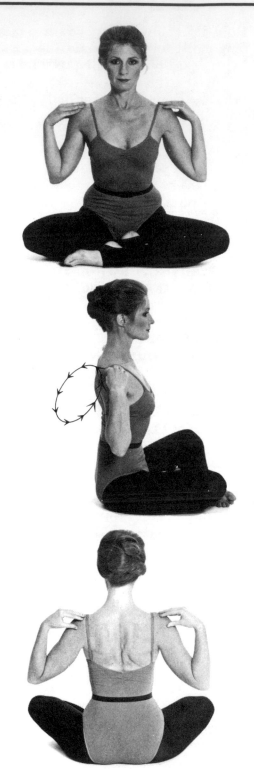

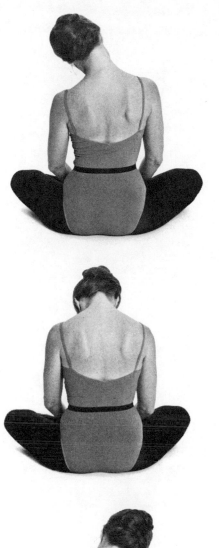

13. HEAD ROLLS—2X EACH SIDE

Purpose
RELAXATION OF NECK MUSCLES
(trapezius, sternomastoid, scaleni).

Position
a. Sit cross-legged on the floor if comfortable; or sit on a chair.
b. Stomach tucked in.
c. Arms relaxed at sides.

Directions
Keep moving smoothly as you
a. Bend left ear to shoulder.
b. Continue down, bending head forward and through to
c. Bend (NOT TURN) right ear to shoulder.
d. Circle back and repeat.

COORDINATE BREATHING
a. Inhale as you begin.
b. Exhale as you drop head forward.
c. Repeat.

Note
Head rolls should be done slowly and smoothly. Be certain to drop shoulders—DON'T HUNCH THEM!

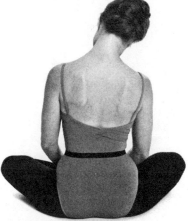

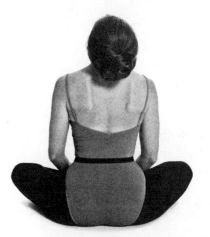

14. FOOT EXERCISES

The concentration of nerve endings in our feet makes them ticklish. But when those nerve endings are irritated, we don't feel like laughing! The following exercises strengthen the arches and are designed to relieve the pressure which causes pain. To do these I prefer to sit on the edge of a pool in the south of France; but a chair or the side of the bed will do.

Note

IT IS IMPORTANT TO KEEP YOUR FEET PARALLEL WHEN YOU DO THESE EXERCISES. If you allow them to turn out, you can weaken your arches.

Directions
a. With legs slightly raised:
   1) Flex feet: stretch heels away, bring toes toward you, then
   2) Point feet.
      • Press down one section of foot at a time:
         —arch (keep toes up)
         —ball of foot (toes still up)
         —top of foot (fill out space on top of foot).
      • Stretch beyond toes.

b. Extend legs straight out in front of you, parallel and a few inches apart.
   1) Keeping heels absolutely still, point toes and imagine them brushing together across a sheet of paper to touch and form an inverted V.
   2) Hold and feel arch in foot pulling up, then relax and *let go*.

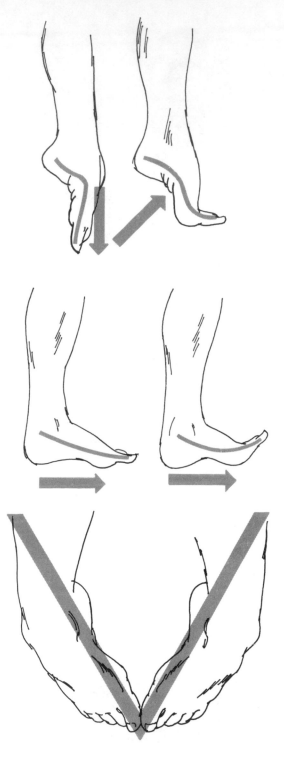

c. Foot circles—for relaxation.
   1) Turn toes in.
   2) Press down through ankles.
   3) Make circles with feet.
d. Curl your toes (the way you make a fist), then spread them wide apart like a fan.
   1) Keep feet parallel and straight.
   2) Repeat three times.
e. Rest feet flat on floor.
   1) Curl toes (like a fist) and feel arches pull up.
   2) Relax.
f. Also:
   1) Place feet on a towel.
   2) Grasp towel with toes and make pleats.

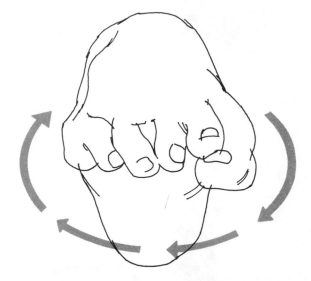

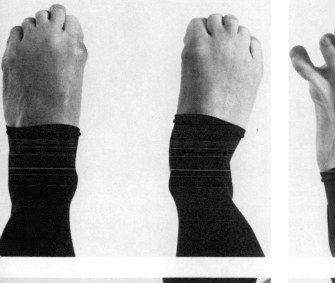

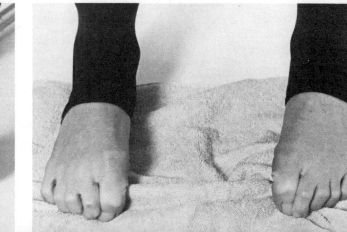

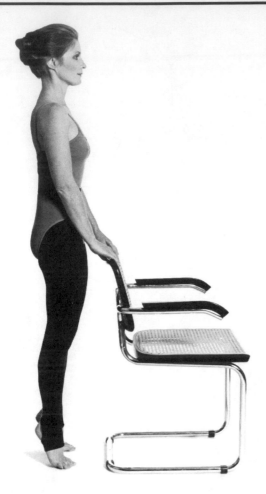

g. To strengthen ankles and stretch calf mucles:
1) Standing, rise slowly up to toes and balls of metatarsals.
2) Lower heels slowly until they touch floor.
3) Repeat.

Now that you've gone through the exercises of Level 1, you've learned the basics of body alignment, stretching and strengthening. In order to get the most from your efforts from the very beginning, I want to urge you to keep these principles in mind during all the nonexercise hours of your day. Transfer your exercises from the floor to your life by taking the following suggestions, which are based on my "Never Do Nothing" outlook on life:

NEVER DO NOTHING EXERCISES

1. Always practice standing in perfect alignment.
   Think of a red traffic light as practice time. If you're standing at a corner, do your whole alignment check. If you're driving, straighten your neck—make that lovely long space between ear and shoulder. Drop shoulders down.

2. Don't stand bored on the bank line—CHECK YOUR SPINE!
   Are your shoulders down?
   Where's your belly? (Tucked in, of course.)
3. Bonus Exercise: Growing on the wall like an ivy vine.
   a. Keep knees bent, feet six inches from wall.
   b. Buttocks against wall, drop head and shoulders.
   c. Let arms dangle loosely and *let go*.
   d. Press belly in as you slowly roll up—lower back straightens
      into wall (keep knees slightly bent).
      Think of pressing one vertebra at a time up against the wall
      as you slowly straighten. Never allow space between your
      lower back and the wall.

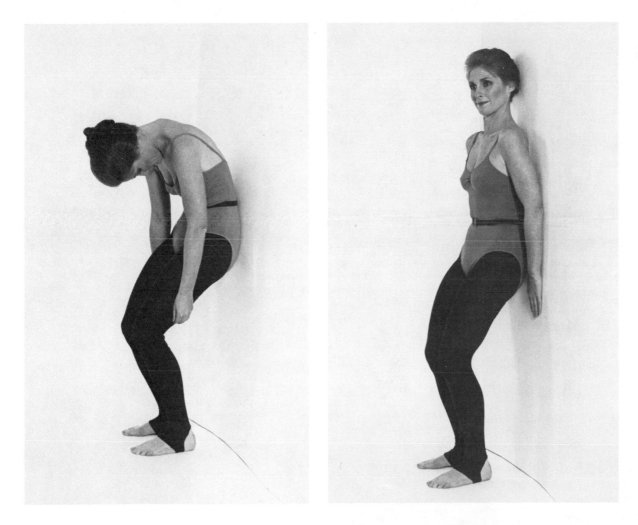

VII

Level 2:
More Variety, Medium-Strong

Arriving at Level 2 means you are now stronger in all areas. Your pain should be gone, and you are ready to continue to develop, safely and sanely—no recurrences of formerly painful conditions and no NEW injuries either. Above all, remember that pain indicates that something you are doing is wrong. If an exercise hurts you, perhaps it is not yet suitable for you. If the exercises of Level 2 cause you pain, continue with Level 1 until you are stronger.

All Level 2 exercises are designed for alignment as much as for stretching and strengthening. Constant awareness of your position makes these exercises productive and keeps them safe. Now you are ready to enlarge your fitness goals. Back pain gone and Level 1 mastered, you can move on to exercises that firm your hips, your thighs and your arms. You are ready to achieve good muscle tone throughout your body WITHOUT HURTING YOUR BACK!

As always, keep repeating the checkpoints to yourself throughout your workout (ankle, knee, hip, shoulder, ear—all in a straight line!). Notice that each exercise level begins with a basic pattern of exercises to loosen muscles so that we can then strengthen them safely and effectively.

1. SIDE SLIDE—3X EACH

Purpose
TO ELIMINATE LOWER-BACK
PAIN—gentle stretching of back muscles to
take pressure off irritated nerves in lower
back.

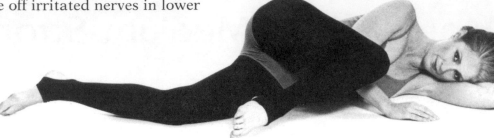

Position
a. Lie comfortably on one side.
b. Gently bend lower leg and rest upper leg
   in space behind knee.
c. Small pillow or lower arm folded under
   head to keep cervical spine straight.
d. Be certain to relax and *let go* of muscles
   in body.

Directions
a. Raise top leg to level of hip.
b. Gently bend knee toward chest, keeping
   at same hip level, and feel back stretch.
c. Slide leg back to starting position—hold
   still and feel weight of leg.
d. Now let leg drop down and *let go*.
   Wobble to loosen body.
e. Repeat (a) through (d) on other side.

Note
Pause between each movement to relax
body. Bend knee toward chest only as high
as is NOT painful. If raising leg to hip level
is painful, *DON'T!!!* Instead, stretch the leg
while resting it on the bent knee, and do the
Side Slide without lifting.

2. PELVIC TILT—5X SLOWLY

Note
In addition to strengthening lower abdominals and tightening transverse as in Level 1, create a total stretch from neck to tailbone by adding the Level 1 neck stretch to this exercise. (Press neck down into floor, as flat as possible.)

Position 1: PELVIC TILT ON BACK
a. Lie on back, knees bent; feet on floor, hip-width apart.

Directions
a. Begin by tensing inner thighs and groin area.
b. Press in lower belly and tighten waist.
c. Press all tummy muscles in toward belly button; with your hands, feel a *concave tummy*.
d. DO NOT HOLD BREATH!
e. Do not lift buttocks, but squeeze together to "set" this position. (Buttocks will automatically lift slightly, and you will feel a tilting up of the pelvis.)
f. Feel for the "cords" at sides of waist; (transverse muscle) feel an east-side to west-side cut along waist; feel a nicely concave tummy.
g. Hold for a slow count of 5—DO NOT HOLD YOUR BREATH—and then *let go*, pause in between and repeat.

Position 2: PELVIC TILT ON STOMACH

a. Lie on stomach; rest forehead on folded hands.

Directions

a. Pinch buttocks together and press down.

b. Pull in transverse and feel tummy lift off floor as back straightens and becomes flat (this is the reverse of the Pelvic Tilt).

c. Keep upper back quiet and DO NOT HOLD BREATH!

Leg Extension

(For people with straight backs, substitute for Pelvic Tilt on Stomach.)

Purpose

TO STRENGTHEN LOWER-BACK MUSCLES AND DEVELOP A HEALTHY CURVE.

Note

DO ONLY IF THERE IS *NO* PAIN.

Position

a. Lie on stomach; rest head on folded hands.

b. Keep upper back quiet.

Directions

a. Keeping hip down, slowly raise single leg (only as high as is comfortable).

b. Put down gently and *let go*.

c. Alternate, three times each leg; when stronger, add double leg lifts, alternating three times.

3. RELAXATION AND ORGANIZATION—
3X EACH

Make these movements part of you so that you will be able to relax and *let go* whenever you need to. Always relax and *let go* between each repetition of a strenuous exercise (or between each irritating phone call of your busy day!).

Purpose
TO ELIMINATE BODY TENSION as in Level 1. Note *new* directions (d) and (e).

Position
a. Lie on back with knees bent; feet flat on floor, hip-width apart.
b. Place hands on belly, let it sink in; and have a concave feeling from ribs down to pubic bone.
c. BACK OF NECK STRETCHED OUT LONG (lots of space between ear and shoulder)—line of sight between knees, not up at ceiling.

Directions

a. Deep breathing—inhale deeply through nose and feel ribs rise. Exhale through mouth and feel ribs lower. Keep inhalation and exhalation time equal. *Let go* and relax before each of the next inhalations. Remember to keep belly in, to move ribs up and down with breathing, and to keep back of neck straight.

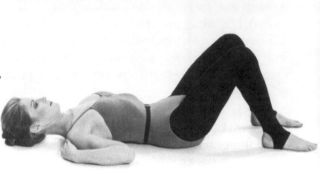

b. Same as (a) with arms stretching UP OVER HEAD on inhalation and dropping straight down one at a time on exhalation.

c. Same as (a) with arms stretching SIDEWAYS up along floor on inhalation, then sideways down on exhalation. Let shoulders and arms wobble on the way down. Keep palms facing toward ceiling as arms sweep up and down.

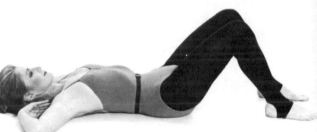

d. Place fingertips on shoulders; wrists and elbows flat to floor.

e. BELLY IN AND NECK STRETCHED, inhale and slide elbows up; exhale and slide elbows down ONLY AS FAR AS ELBOWS AND WRISTS STAY FLAT ON FLOOR.

f. Check your alignment!

g. Wobble head to loosen.

h. Wobble shoulders to loosen.

i. Keep heels on floor as you let each leg slide down slowly; slide until you can *let go* and drop leg. Wobble legs and *let go* of muscles.

Note

REPEAT HEAD AND SHOULDER WOBBLES THROUGHOUT WORKOUT. The neck and shoulder area is the likeliest spot for tension to accumulate.

4. NECK ROTATION—1X EACH SIDE

Purpose
TO STRENGTHEN MUSCLES IN NECK as you use them to support weight of head.

Position
a. Tummy in, neck straight.
b. Slide back of neck as straight down into floor as possible (chin will go down as head bends forward).
c. Prepare to use right hand at back of neck to guide rotation to left; use left hand to guide right rotation. (When you are stronger and can hold position correctly, NO HANDS.)

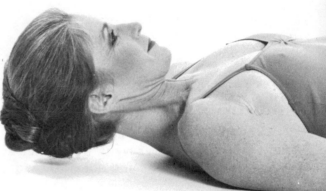

Directions
a. Bend head forward and only slightly off mat.
b. Use back of neck to hold weight of head; turn head slowly and look over left shoulder, keeping back of neck straight, shoulders down.
c. Come to center (rest, if tired) and repeat to other side. Do the rotation without rest only if you can keep neck in position without tensing front of neck and jaw.

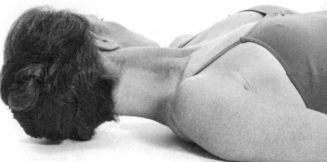

Note
As you turn to the side, feel strong cords up and down sides of neck (sternomastoid muscle) strengthening. ONLY DO ROTATION WITHOUT HANDS WHEN YOU ARE STRONG ENOUGH TO MAINTAIN CORRECT STRETCHED POSITION WITH *CHIN DOWN*.

5. CROSSOVER SPINE STRETCH— ALTERNATE 3X EACH SIDE

Purpose
TO RELAX BACK MUSCLES—to eliminate feeling of stiffness in back.

Position:
a. Lie on back, knees bent and feet on floor.
b. Arms at sides OR folded beneath head.

Directions
a. Stretch left leg toward ceiling and keep knee softly bent for comfort, foot loose.
b. Cross left leg over right (bent) knee and stretch body over and down toward right.

c. Feel a pleasant stretch in back; keep shoulders reasonably flat and down; elbows too; loosen and stretch neck muscles while in this position.
d. To return: Pull left leg back up to ceiling by tensing inner thighs and pressing belly in. Keep shoulders quiet.

e. Bend left leg and repeat on right side
and/or
a. Lie on back, legs straight.
b. Arms out to sides or folded beneath
head.

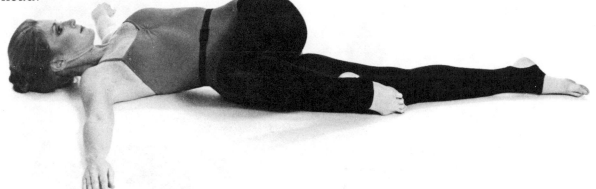

c. Bend left knee and place foot on flat
right thigh.
d. Stretch legs over and down toward right
keeping shoulders quietly down.
e. Inhale and return to starting position.
(To return: tense inner thighs and
abdominal muscles.)
f. Drop left leg down and repeat, other
side.

Note
Substitute Level 1 Knee Hug (No. 5) to
stretch lower back muscles if **Spine Stretch**
is not comfortable.

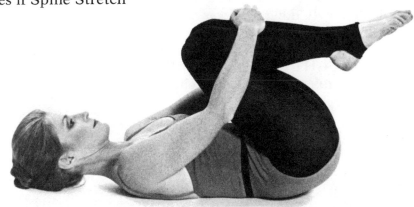

6. OPPOSITE ELBOW TO KNEE STRETCH—ALTERNATE 3X EACH SIDE

Purpose
TO STRENGTHEN DIAGONAL OBLIQUE
MUSCLES IN ABDOMEN.

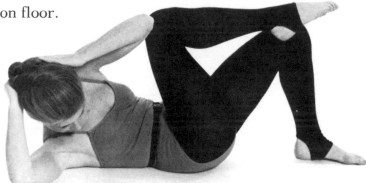

Position
a. Lie on back, knees bent; feet on floor.
b. Arms folded under head.

Directions
a. Raise right knee (foot pointed) and left elbow.
b. Touch elbow to outside of knee.
c. Hold and "set" your muscles: look under right arm and press belly in very hard (feel diagonal muscles tightening).
d. Roll slowly down to floor.
   Note
   be aware of alignment; PULL UP THROUGH CENTER OF BODY—ankles, knees, inner thighs, pelvis, chest, neck.
e. Repeat, other side.

Coordinate Breathing
a. Inhale to begin.
b. Exhale on way up.
c. Breathe normally and concentrate on "setting" muscles on way down.

7. ALTERNATE LEG STRETCH— 10X, ALTERNATING LEGS

Purpose
TO STRENGTHEN ABDOMINALS AND TO STRETCH HAMSTRINGS. (Note: because muscles work in corresponding pairs, when you strengthen abdominals, you also loosen and stretch back muscles.)

Position
a. Lie on back, legs down flat.
b. Arms at sides.
c. Feet pointed, belly in, back of neck stretched.

Directions
a. Bend left knee to chest, left hand holding ankle and right hand holding knee.
b. Lift head and shoulders. (Let entire upper back hold weight of head so neck does not strain.)
c. Bend head forward to stretch cervical spine (neck).
d. Raise right leg two inches up from floor as you hold position.
e. Squeeze muscles in, hold and "set," and
f. Change sides—outside hand always on ankle, inside hand always on knee. DO NOT HUNCH SHOULDERS AND NECK.

Coordinate Breathing
a. Inhale when you change sides.
b. Exhale when you "set" muscles.

8. HAMSTRING STRETCH II— 3X EACH LEG

Purpose
TO STRETCH HAMSTRINGS GRACEFULLY. (Enjoy making the movements pretty.)

Position
a. Lie on back, knees bent; feet on floor.
b. Arms at sides.
c. Belly in and neck stretched. (Check your alignment and be aware of it throughout exercise.)

Directions
a. Work one leg at a time, keeping opposite knee bent; drop right leg down.
b. Flex right foot to stretch leg and check alignment.
c. Point right foot and raise leg two inches up from floor.
d. Bend knee to chest, KEEPING BUTTOCKS *DOWN*.
e. Flex foot, pause, and "set" muscles.
f. Stretch leg up toward ceiling—let heel pull leg up; stretch leg ONLY as high as knee stays straight (but not locked and rigid).

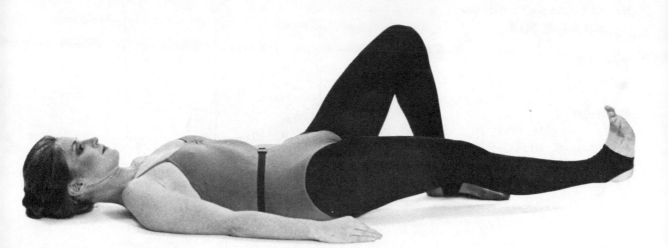

g. Slowly lower straight leg to two inches up from floor. (Remember to pull up through center of body, starting from ankle, as straight leg lowers. Keep stretching heel. Feel stretch on back of leg.)

h. Point foot and repeat, two more times; drop leg on last repetition, bend that knee, and

i. Repeat, other side.

Coordinate Breathing

a. Inhale as you begin and bend knee to chest.

b. Exhale as you stretch heel up to ceiling.

c. Breathe normally throughout.

9. LEG LIFTS ON SIDE— 8X EACH SIDE

Purpose
TO TIGHTEN *LOWER* BELLY.

Position
a. Lie on side, body in a completely straight line (CHECKPOINTS: ear, shoulder, hip, knee, ankle).
b. Bend elbow to support head in hand.

Directions
The directions that follow are the same as for the Level 1 Leg Lifts, but you should increase the feeeling of resistance and tension between legs as you raise and lower. The heavier you make the leg, the stronger the abdominals become. Repeat checkpoints on each lift. ALWAYS KEEP BELLY IN TO PROTECT BACK.
a. Tighten transverse before each leg lift.
b. SLOWLY raise leg straight up and down (with resistance* to increase difficulty) as you
c. Keep knee forward—don't let it turn up toward ceiling; pull up through center of body as you lower leg.
d. Keep hip rotated in—this tightens buttocks.
e. Allow NO sway in body—the tighter you hold your belly, the less you move.
f. Hold weight of leg by tightening lower belly.

Coordinate Breathing
a. Breathe in to begin.
b. Exhale as you slowly stretch leg up.
c. Inhale just after you lower.

*Resistance

a. As you raise, think of heavy weight on top of leg; press against heavy weight.

b. As you lower, think of pressing down against heavy metal bar.

c. Think of magnetic pull between inner thighs, and keep turning leg in.

10. ONE-LEGGED CURL-BACKS— 3X EACH SIDE

Purpose

TO STRENGTHEN ABDOMINALS in a more strenuous way than in Level 1.

Position

a. Sit with one knee bent, foot on floor close to buttocks; other leg straight out on floor.

b. Point straight-leg foot hard; keep bent-leg foot down throughout exercise.

c. Head bent forward and arms loose at sides.

Directions

a. Roll slowly back down toward floor.

b. Stop just before waist touches floor (or before feet start to lift up).

c. Hold and "set" muscles: press head down; press all muscles in belly toward belly button; keep feet down.

d. Pull forward to sitting: press in belly even harder to lift ribs; pull up through center of legs and pelvis and up to center of abdomen. Join the abdominal pull at your belly button!

Coordinate Breathing

a. Inhale to help pull you forward.

b. Exhale on roll-down as you press in abdominals.

To Increase Difficulty

As you hold and "set" muscles (see step c above under Directions, page 77), eliminate help given by arms and shoulders:

a. Bring arms straight forward; *let go* in shoulders; use strength from abdominals to hold position; KEEP FEET DOWN.

b. Reach arms up and cross them behind head; keep squeezing in.

c. Raise crossed arms up and bring them forward; drop and *let go*.

d. Pull forward to sitting; lean to each side to loosen muscles before next repetition.

11. HIP ROLLS—
ALTERNATE 3X EACH SIDE

Purpose
TO STRENGTHEN ABDOMINALS—to
firm hips and thighs.

Position
a. Lie on back, knees together and bent on
   chest.
b. Arms out sideways, a bit lower than
   shoulders; palms up.

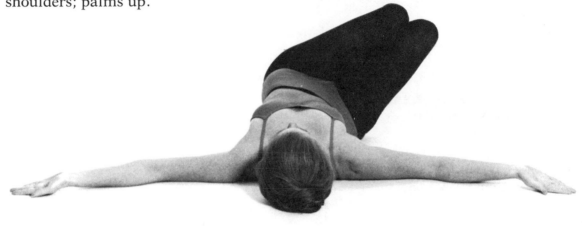

Directions
a. Stretch knees toward right only as far as
   is comfortable; only as far as shoulders
   stay down flat.
b. Keep feet pointed, knees pressed
   together.
c. Squeeze belly in hard and use transverse
   particularly to pull knees back to center.
d. Keep belly in, shoulders down, neck
   straight, and
e. Repeat to other side.

Coordinate Breathing
a. Inhale to bring knees to center.
b. Exhale as you stretch to side.

12. KNEE-HEEL SITTING

This is a position rather than an exercise. Use it for relaxation; or to connect two exercises smoothly (*e.g.*, from Hip Rolls, above, to Round Back–Flat Back, next).

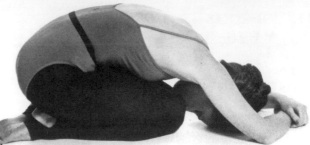

Directions

a. Put knees on floor and sit on heels.

b. Head and shoulders drop down toward floor.

c. Stretch from under buttocks, press in belly and feel long muscles on back lengthen and relax.

d. Sway from side to side and *let go* of all muscles.

13. ROUND BACK–FLAT BACK— 3X EACH POSITION

Purpose

TO STRETCH BACK MUSCLES AND TIGHTEN ABDOMINALS.

Note

Be especially aware of alignment as you do this exercise. Perfect alignment will become a habit sooner, the more you practice it in all positions.

Position

Begin on hands and knees, arms straight and belly in.

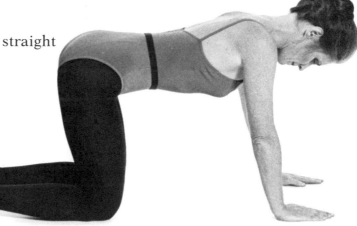

Directions

a. Make back as flat as table.

b. Squeeze transverse muscle in tightly.

c. Drop between shoulder blades to eliminate hunching; keep neck same height as back.

d. Keep spine straight, from tailbone up to head.

e. Pull head down, press in belly and make back round. (Have you ever seen a frightened cat round its back up in alarm?)

f. Hold in hard: inner thighs, buttocks and abdominals—as you

g. Lift tailbone and return to Flat Back position   and/or

a. As you ROUND back, bring right knee to forehead.

b. Stretch right leg straight back on same level as back, as you FLATTEN back.

Coordinate Breathing

a. Inhale as you flatten back.

b. Exhale as you round back. (Exhaling helps you to tighten abdominals.)

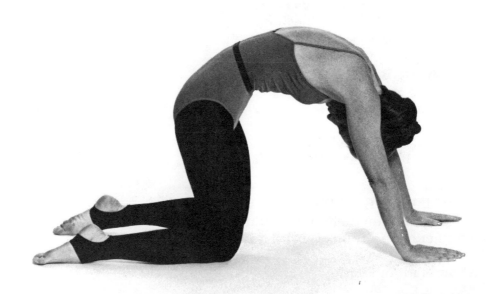

14. CAT STRETCH—3X

Purpose
TO STRETCH PECTORAL MUSCLES (on chest).

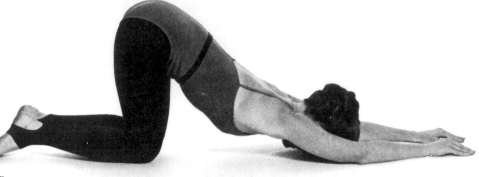

Position
a. Knee-heel sitting.
b. Forehead down and arms straight out on floor.

Directions
a. Raise hips high, in line with knees, as you
b. Slide chest and arms forward; KEEP HIPS STILL.
c. Sink down across upper back and try to place forehead on floor.
d. Do not arch back.
e. Press chest gently down; feel a comfortable stretch in arms.
f. Return to knee-heel position.
g. Wobble and loosen body.

Coordinate Breathing
a. Inhale as you raise hips.
b. Exhale as you stretch forward.

15. SHOULDER CIRCLES— 5X SLOWLY AND CORRECTLY

Purpose
TO ELIMINATE UPPER BACK AND NECK PAIN—to eliminate round shoulders by lengthening pectoral muscles; to tighten muscles that hold shoulder blades and spine (rhomboid muscles).

Note

It's easy to do this exercise completely ineffectually. It can look right, but it won't do you any good unless you feel a specific tightening *between* shoulder bladers. BE CERTAIN TO RELAX AND *LET GO* BETWEEN EACH STEP: Try shoulder shrugs, head rolls, deep breathing. (Directions for head rolls follow this exercise).

Position

a. Sit cross-legged on the floor if comfortable; or sit on a chair.
b. Belly tucked in.
c. Chest in front of stomach—keep weight forward.
d. Back of neck straight; back of head in line with upper back; chin level.
e. Shoulders relaxed and down—nice big open space between ear and shoulder.

Directions

a. Bend arms and place fingertips on shoulders.
b. Slowly make backward circles.

Note

This movement is done by shoulder, *not* elbow; so check that shoulder stays farther *back* than elbow.

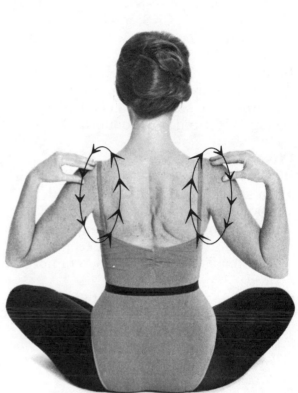

1) Begin with a slight lift.
2) Keep circling motion behind you.
3) Slowly roll all the way back.
4) Feel shoulder blades come together and blend movement to
5) Pull down, keeping shoulders *back* (the movement is both back and down).
6) *Let go*, and return to starting position.
7) PAUSE, and repeat.

16. SITTING RELAXATION

Purpose
TO KEEP SPINE FLEXIBLE—to loosen
back muscles and tighten abdominals.

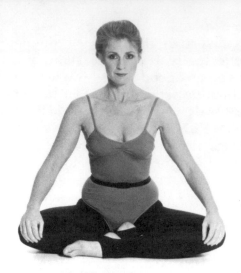

Position
a. Sit cross-legged—NEVER SLUMP BACK
   INTO BUTTOCKS; always reach
   forward from under tailbone; arms
   loosely at sides.
b. Use pillow under back half of buttocks if
   muscles are too stiff to sit forward.
c. Substitute sitting in a chair if cross-
   legged sitting is uncomfortable.

Directions
BODY ROLL—2 or 3X in each direction
a. In a loose and flexible manner, lean
   shoulders and ribs to left.
b. Circle down to left knee, and
c. Continue through center, keeping chest
   and head as low to floor as comfortable,
   and
d. Continue through to right knee.
e. Squeeze in waist and pull up through
   center of body to lift.
   1) Squeeze both inner thighs.
   2) Pull up through center of pelvis.
   3) Through center of chest.
   4) Lift ribs.
   5) Let back of neck pull you up.
   6) Drop shoulders.

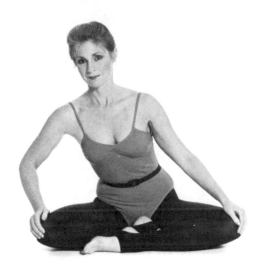

Check
a. Alignment: see that center of pelvis is in
   line with chest and with head.
b. Belly tight, back loose.
c. Chest more prominent than belly.
d. Sit forward on "sit bones"—don't sink
   back.

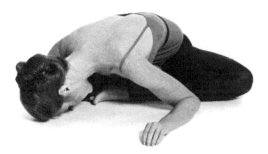

HEAD ROLL—2 or 3 X in each direction
a. Bend left ear to shoulder and circle head down.
b. Rest chin on chest and feel stretch in cervical spine.
c. Continue circle and bend right ear to shoulder.
d. Finish circle by rolling head all the way back.
e. Keep shoulders quiet and down throughout; keep body weight forward.

Coordinate Breathing
For both Body and Head Rolls
a. Inhale as you start to roll.
b. Exhale as you continue Head Roll.
c. Exhale as you circle down to floor for Body Roll; inhale to help you lift up.

SIDE BENDS—alternate 3X each side
a. Sit cross-legged and check alignment (both hips MUST stay down).
b. Stretch right arm up overhead; turn palm to face ceiling.
c. Bend body sideways to left—only as far as hips stay down; feel stretch in waist.
d. Squeeze belly in and pull up through center of body to lift you up—DO NOT USE ARM TO LIFT BODY!!! Let back of neck pull you up.
e. When you are up, separate space between ear and shoulder: 1) Stretch back of neck as long as possible; 2) drop shoulders down as low as possible.
f. Repeat, other side.

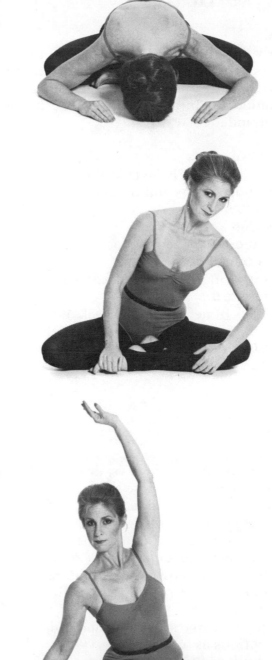

17. ARM EXERCISES

Note
Only do this series after your pectoral (chest) muscles are sufficiently stretched: you must be able to sit straight with shoulders pointing to ceiling, NOT hunched or rounded forward.

Purpose
TO FIRM UPPER AND LOWER ARMS (deltoids, biceps and triceps).

Position
a. Sit cross-legged on floor.
b. Stomach tucked in.
c. Chest in front of stomach; weight forward.
d. Back of neck straight; back of head in line with upper back; chin level.
e. Shoulders relaxed and down—a nice big open space between ear and shoulder.

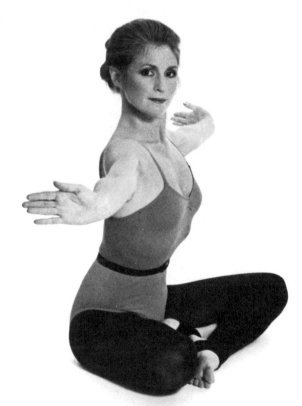

Directions
a. Stretch arms sideways; drop shoulders.
b. Flex hands and raise them slightly higher than shoulders.
c. Press shoulder blades together as you pulse wrists farther and farther away to the sides and slightly back (5X).
d. Turn palms down, circle thumbs under and back until palms face ceiling ''backwards.''
e. Repeat same stretching and pulsing motions as (c) above.
f. Check position: shoulders point to ceiling; hands slightly higher than shoulders; shoulders DOWN; neck long and stretched.

g. RELAXATION:
  1) Arms loosely at sides.
  2) Stretch from under buttocks.
  3) Press in belly, drop head and shoulders toward floor and stretch back muscles.

18. RELAXATION AND ORGANIZATION

Position
a. Lie on back, knees bent; feet on floor.

Directions
From Exercise 3, Level 2, select assorted breathing, wobbling. *LET GO* all of the tension in your body.

19. SIDE SLIDE—3X EACH SIDE
ALWAYS TRY TO BEGIN AND END WITH THIS EXERCISE.

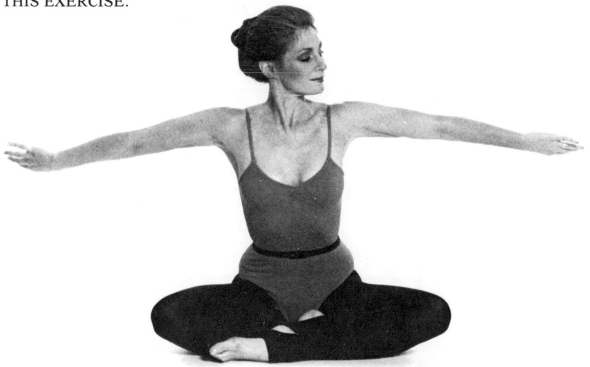

VIII

Level 3:
Aesthetic and Strong

The purpose of Level 1 was training—you learned about your body structure and alignment. Level 2 was designed to stretch and strengthen you from head to toe. Our purpose here in Level 3 is more aesthetic than it could have been before. Until now you've worked reclining on your mat. We attended to your trunk to give you a firm foundation. Now you will stand up to expand your movement vocabulary.

The third level of the Back in Shape program introduces you to more strenuous exercises. By now you should have the strength to do them safely. Our goal here is to firm your hips and thighs. But a word of caution first: Legs are heavy. *Without* strong abdominals to support their weight you are in *danger* of straining your back. By Level 3 you should have achieved that level of strength. If you remember to stay within your comfort range, if you always pay attention to how you feel, you will avoid injury!

Having acquired the essential equipment of knowledge and strength, you can now build a more beautiful body, a body that will please you in the mirror as well as in comfort, relaxation and strength. Of course, I will not turn you loose to work without my favorite reminder: CHECKPOINTS FIRST AND THROUGHOUT.

1. SIDE SLIDE—3X EACH

Purpose
TO ELIMINATE LOWER-BACK
PAIN—gentle stretching of back muscles to
take pressure off irritated nerves in lower
back.

Position
a. Lie comfortably on one side.
b. Gently bend lower leg and rest upper leg
in space behind knee.
c. Small pillow or lower arm folded under
head to keep cervical spine straight.
d. Be certain to relax and *let go* of muscles
in body.

Directions
a. Raise top leg to level of hip.
b. Gently bend knee toward chest, keeping
at same hip level, and feel back stretch.
c. Slide leg back to starting position—hold
still and feel weight of leg.
d. Now let leg drop down and *let go*.
Wobble to loosen body.
e. Repeat (a) through (d) on other side.

Note
Pause between each movement to relax
body. Bend knee toward chest only as high
as is NOT painful. If raising leg to hip level
is painful, DON'T! Instead, stretch the leg
while resting it on the bent knee, and do the
Side Slide without lifting.

2.   PELVIC TILT—5X SLOWLY

Purpose
TO STRENGTHEN LOWER ABDOMINALS
AND TIGHTEN TRANSVERSE—to create
total stretch from neck to tailbone.

Position
a. Lie on back, knees bent; feet on floor,
     hip-width apart.
b. Press neck down into floor, as flat as
     possible.

Directions
a. Begin by tensing inner thighs and groin
     area.
b. Press in lower belly and tighten waist.
c. Press all tummy muscles in toward belly
     button; with your hands, feel a *concave*
     tummy.
d. DO NOT HOLD BREATH!
e. Do not lift buttocks, but squeeze
     together to "set" this position. (Buttocks
     will automatically lift slightly, and you
     will feel a tilting up of pelvis.)
f. Feel for "cords" at sides of waist; feel an
     east-side to west-side cut along waist;
     feel a nicely concave tummy.
g. Hold for a slow count of 5—DO NOT
     HOLD YOUR BREATH—and then *let go*,
     pause in between and repeat.

Note
For Pelvic Tilt on Stomach and Leg
Extension, see Level 1, No. 3.

3. RELAXATION AND ORGANIZATION—
3X EACH

Make these movements part of you so that
you will be able to relax and *let go* whenever
you need to. Always relax and *let go* between
each repetition of a strenuous exercise.

Purpose

TO ELIMINATE BODY TENSION as in
Level 1. Note *new* directions (d) and (e).

Position

a. Lie on back with knees bent; feet flat on
   floor, hip-width apart.
b. Place hands on belly, let it sink in; and
   have a concave feeling from ribs down to
   pubic bone.
c. BACK OF NECK STRETCHED OUT
   LONG (lots of space between ear and
   shoulder)—line of sight between knees,
   not up at ceiling.

Directions

a. Deep breathing—inhale deeply through nose and feel ribs rise. Exhale through mouth and feel ribs lower. Keep inhalation and exhalation time equal. *Let go* and relax before each of the next inhalations. Remember to keep belly in, to move ribs up and down with breathing, and to keep back of neck straight.

b. Same as (a) with arms stretching UP OVER HEAD on inhalation and dropping straight down one at a time on exhalation.

c. Same as (a) with arms stretching SIDEWAYS up along floor on inhalation, then sideways down on exhalation. Let shoulders and arms wobble on the way down. Keep palms facing toward ceiling as arms sweep up and down.

d. Place fingertips on shoulders; wrists and elbows flat to floor.

e. BELLY IN AND NECK STRETCHED, inhale and slide elbows up; exhale and slide elbows down ONLY AS FAR AS ELBOWS AND WRISTS STAY FLAT ON FLOOR.

f. Check your alignment!

g. Wobble head to loosen.

h. Wobble shoulders to loosen.

i. Keep heels on floor as you let each leg slide down slowly; slide until you can *let go* and drop leg. Wobble legs and *let go* of muscles.

Note

REPEAT HEAD AND SHOULDER WOBBLES THROUGHOUT WORKOUT. The neck and shoulder area is the likeliest spot for tension to accumulate.

4A. ACCORDION NECK STRETCH—
3X EACH

Purpose
TO ELIMINATE NECK PAIN—to lengthen
and strengthen the trapezius muscle, which
keeps the cervical spine straight.

Position
a. Lie on back, knees bent; feet on floor,
hip-width apart.
b. Small pillow or folded towel under neck
if necessary for comfort.
c. ORGANIZE YOURSELF—start each
movement with "My belly in and my
neck straight. . . ."

Directions
NECK STRETCH *WITH* HANDS
a. Put hands out in front of you and bend
elbows.
b. Hold on to back of head at top.
c. Pull head forward slightly off mat and
stretch cervical spine (back of neck).
d. Carefully place down seventh
cervical—the bump at top of
spine—then, one vertebra at a time,
lower until head is flat down, cervical
spine as straight as comfortable. (Use
pillow under head to "raise floor" until
muscle becomes stretched enough to
reach floor by itself.)
NECK STRETCH *WITHOUT* HANDS
a. Tummy in, neck straight.
b. Slide back of neck as straight down into
floor as possible (chin will go down as
head bends forward). DO NOT LIFT!
Feel back of neck stretch and elongate.
Imagine a sponge underneath neck;
imagine pressing sponge down into floor.
Press, pause; press, pause. Always
wobble to loosen.

4B. NECK ROTATION— 3X EACH SIDE

Purpose
TO STRENGTHEN MUSCLES IN NECK as you use them to support weight of head.

Position
a. Tummy in, neck straight.
b. Slide back of neck as straight down into floor as possible (chin will go down as head bends forward).
c. Prepare to use right hand at back of neck to guide rotation to left; use left hand to guide right rotation. (When you are stronger and can hold position correctly, NO HANDS.)

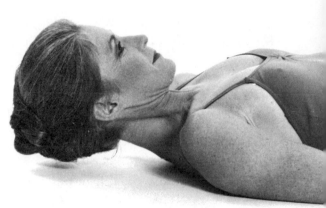

Directions
a. Bend head forward and only slightly off mat.
b. Use back of neck to hold weight of head; turn head slowly and look over left shoulder, keeping back of neck straight, shoulders down.
c. Come to center (rest, if tired) and repeat to other side. Do the rotation without rest only if you can keep neck in position without tensing front of neck and jaw.

Note
As you turn to the side, feel strong cords up and down sides of neck (sternomastoid muscle) strengthening. ONLY DO ROTATION WITHOUT HANDS WHEN YOU ARE STRONG ENOUGH TO MAINTAIN CORRECT STRETCHED POSITION WITH *CHIN DOWN*.

5. CROSSOVER SPINE STRETCH— ALTERNATE 3X EACH SIDE

Purpose
TO RELAX BACK MUSCLES—to eliminate feeling of stiffness in back.

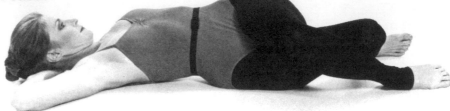

Position
a. Lie on back, knees bent and feet on floor.
b. Arms at sides OR folded beneath head.

Directions
a. Stretch left leg toward ceiling and keep knee softly bent for comfort, foot loose.
b. Cross left leg over right (bent) knee and stretch body over and down toward right.
c. Feel a pleasant stretch in back; keep shoulders reasonably flat and down; elbows too; loosen and stretch neck muscles while in this position.
d. To return: Pull left leg back up to ceiling by tensing inner thighs and pressing belly in. Keep shoulders quiet.
e. Bend left leg and repeat on right side
                    and/or
a. Lie on back, legs straight.
b. Arms out to sides or folded beneath head.
c. Bend left knee and place foot on flat right thigh.
d. Stretch legs over and down toward right keeping shoulders quietly down.
e. Inhale and return to starting position. (To return: tense inner thighs and abdominal muscles.)
f. Drop left leg down and repeat, other side.

Note
Substitute Level 1 Knee Hug (No. 5) to
stretch lower back muscles if Spine Stretch
is not comfortable.

6. OPPOSITE ELBOW TO KNEE STRETCH— 10X ALTERNATING LEGS

Purpose
TO STRENGTHEN DIAGONAL OBLIQUE
MUSCLES IN ABDOMEN.

Position
a. Lie on back, legs STRAIGHT, feet
   pointed.
b. Arms folded under head.

Directions
a. Lift head and shoulders; bring right knee
   (foot pointed) to chest and touch
   opposite (left) elbow to (right) knee.
b. Touch elbow to outside of knee.
c. Straight leg is raised two inches up from
   floor.
d. Hold and "set" muscles: look under right
   arm and press belly in very hard (feel
   diagonal muscles tightening).
e. Repeat, other side.
   Note: Be aware of alignment; PULL UP
   THROUGH CENTER OF BODY—ankles,
   knees, inner thighs, pelvis, chest, neck.

Coordinate Breathing
a. Inhale on change of sides.
b. Exhale when you hold and "set"
   muscles.

7. LEG LIFTS ON SIDE—10X

Hold the level of tension in leg and lower abdomen (to keep exercise effective). The number of lifts is not important: *how thoroughly and correctly you do them determines how much benefit you get from all exercises.*

Purpose
TO TIGHTEN LOWER BELLY.

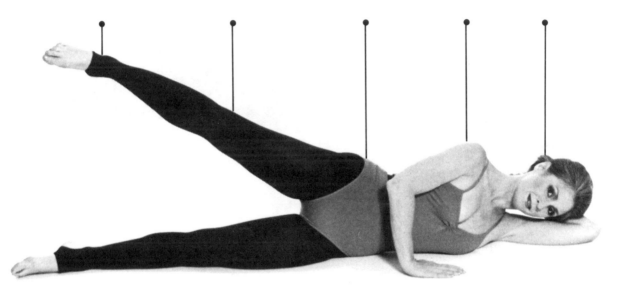

Position
a. Lie on side, body in a completely straight line (CHECKPOINTS: ear, shoulder, hip, knee, ankle).
b. Bend elbow to support head in hand.

Directions

The directions which follow are the same as for the Level 1 Leg Lifts, but you should increase the feeling of resistance and tension between legs as you raise and lower. The heavier you make the leg, the stronger the abdominals become. Repeat checkpoints on each lift. ALWAYS KEEP BELLY IN TO PROTECT BACK.

a. Tighten transverse before each leg lift.
b. SLOWLY raise leg straight up and down. (with resistance to increase difficulty) as you
c. Keep knee forward—don't let it turn up toward ceiling; pull up through center of body as you lower leg.
d. Keep hip rotated in—this tightens buttocks.
e. Allow NO sway in body—the tighter you hold your belly, the less you move.
f. Hold weight of leg by tightening lower belly.

Coordinate Breathing

a. Breathe in to begin.
b. Exhale as you slowly stretch leg up.
c. Inhale just after you lower.

8. THREE-LEVEL LEG STRETCH— ALTERNATE 3X EACH LEG

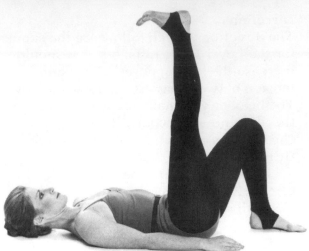

Purpose
TO LENGTHEN HAMSTRINGS AND TIGHTEN ABDOMINALS.

Position
a. Lie on back, knees bent; feet on floor.
b. Arms at sides.

Directions
a. Be aware of checkpoints—keep belly in and back of neck straight; make sure NOT to lift buttocks each time you stretch leg.

Level 1
b. Bring right knee to chest; flex foot and stretch leg straight up toward ceiling.

Level 2
c. Bend knee to chest; keep foot flexed and stretch leg straight out, halfway down to floor.

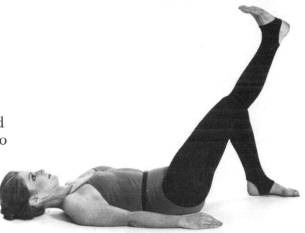

Level 3
d. Bend knee to chest; keep foot flexed and stretch leg out parallel to floor, two inches up.
e. Bend knee to chest; put foot down; drop leg down; *let go* and relax.
f. Repeat with left leg; always keep opposite knee bent.

OR
BONUS HAMSTRING STRETCH

a. Bring left knee to chest; stretch leg straight up to ceiling, foot pointed.
b. Lift head and shoulders (use upper back to hold weight of head); hug leg with hands and pull toward you; feel stretch behind knee.
c. Keep head bent forward with chin resting on chest.
d. Flex foot and, keeping leg up, bend knee toward shoulder.
e. Keep leg as close to you as you can and slowly stretch straight up.
f. Bend knee to chest; drop foot to floor; drop leg down to *let go* and relax.
g. Repeat, other side; always keep opposite knee bent.

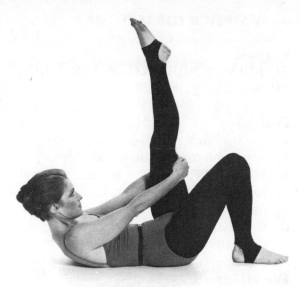

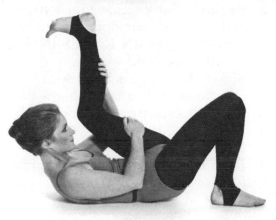

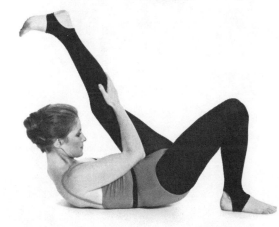

9. V STRETCH FOR LEGS—3X

Purpose
TO FIRM INNER AND OUTER THIGH
MUSCLES.

Position
a. Lie on back, knees to chest.
b. Arms diagonally down at sides.
c. TO START: Squeeze knees and thighs
   together; feet wide apart and parallel to
   floor.
d. Belly in; neck straight and long;
   shoulders quiet and down.

Directions
a. Beginning at knees, against strong
   resistance, slowly open legs to ceiling in
   V position; TURN KNEES IN; keep feet
   pointed and hold.
b. Slowly bend knees back down; continue
   resistance and squeeze thighs together.
c. Return to starting position and hold.
d. Repeat two times.
e. Release and *let go*.
f. Bend knees to chest; softly bounce loose
   feet toward bottom.

10. GRADED SIT-UPS—BEGIN WITH 3X
AND BUILD UP TO 10X

Note
All the muscles in the body except those of the lower back aid us in doing straight-leg sit-ups. When done correctly—by CURLING UP and ALWAYS KEEPING THE BELLY IN—they are safe and effective. If done incorrectly—by tightening the back muscles rather than the abdominals—you will irritate nerves in your back. **Please follow the directions carefully in order to avoid irritation.** If the straight-leg sit-up is uncomfortable, substitute the bent-knee position also listed below. Bent knees eliminate aid from the rest of your muscles, so you may need to use a heavy weight across your feet to accomplish the exercise in this position.

If the bent-knee sit-up is also uncomfortable, substitute the Curl-Back and Diagonal Curl-Back from Level 1.

Purpose
TO TIGHTEN AND STRENGTHEN ABDOMINAL MUSCLES and thereby take pressure off lower back. (This group will make you look wonderful and feel a great sense of accomplishment.)

Position
a. Lie on back, legs straight. (If abdominal muscles are weak and you need extra help, place weight across feet to keep them down.)
    or
    If (a) causes discomfort,
b. Lie on back, knees bent; feet on floor (plus an even heavier weight).
c. ALWAYS KEEP WAIST PULLED IN TIGHT TO PROTECT LOWER BACK MUSCLES.

Directions: Basic Sit-Up

Arms overhead

a. Swing arms forward; use momentum of swing to pull you up; keep chin tucked in.

b. Let neck and upper back muscles lift head off floor; then squeeze belly in HARD to pull ribs off floor and sit up.

c. Pull waist in to keep strain from lower back.

d. Sit straight; knees softly bent.

e. CHECK ALIGNMENT—is trunk in straight line with pelvis? Remember checkpoints: hip, shoulder, ear.

f. Roll down slowly, back rounded and belly pulled in.

Arms at sides: MORE DIFFICULT

a. Lift head to begin.

b. Bend head forward, chin in, then shoulders.

c. Pull waist in to keep strain from lower back.

d. Roll up and sit straight, knees softly bent.

e. Roll down slowly, back rounded and belly IN.

Arms folded across chest: another more difficult sit-up; follow steps (a) through (e) of previous sit-up.

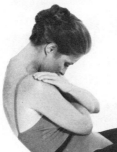

Hands behind neck: DIFFICULT
a. Keep elbows straight out to sides.
b. Follow steps (a) through (e) as in previous sit-up.

Coordinate Breathing
a. Inhale before you begin.
b. Exhale as you roll up.
c. Breathe in and out as you sit straight and lift ribs.
d. Exhale as you curl down.

Note
What makes the previous three sit-ups more difficult than the Basic Sit-Up is that you get less help from your arms.

11. MIRACULOUS HIP AND THIGH TIGHTENERS
4X INCREASING TO 8X AS YOU GROW STRONGER

Purpose
TO FIRM HIPS AND THIGHS AND
ELIMINATE "SADDLE BAGS" ON HIPS.

Position
a. Lie on side in perfectly straight
   alignment, both legs straight (you may
   keep lower leg bent slightly back at first
   if more comfortable).
b. Bend bottom arm; lift head and rest in
   hand.
c. Keep belly in to protect back and to keep
   hip still. DO NOT MOVE HIP, move leg!
d. Keep hips in straight line.

Directions
a. Flex upper foot; rotate and turn knee in
   and lift top leg slightly higher than hip.
b. Stretch heel as far away as possible, as
   you bounce leg four times lightly—KEEP
   KNEE TURNED IN.
c. Holding flexed and turned-in position,
   move leg slightly behind you.
d. Trace little circles with foot—four
   backward first, then four forward—NO
   MOVEMENT IN BODY OTHER THAN
   LEG—keep stretching heel away.
e. Belly in, hip straight and still.
f. Hold starting position and move leg
   slightly in front of you; repeat circles.
g. Start with these directions and when
   you are stronger, add two higher levels
   at which you do bounces and circles.
   1) Mid-level lift.
   2) Highest leg-lift level at which you can
      hold the starting flexed, turned-in
      position.

Note
To make this exercise super-effective, keep
stretching heel farther and farther away
from you; leg as straight and turned in as
possible.

12. CAT STRETCH—3X

Purpose
TO STRETCH PECTORAL MUSCLES (on
chest). **Note:** This is the same exercise as
Cat Stretch, Level 2, No. 14.

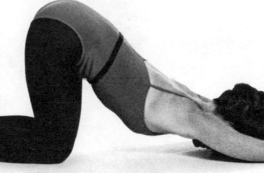

Position
a. Knee-heel sitting.
b. Forehead down and arms straight out on
floor.

Directions
a. Raise hips high, in line with knees, as
you
b. Slide chest and arms forward; KEEP
HIPS STILL.
c. Sink down across upper back and try to
place forehead on floor.
d. Do not arch back.
e. Press chest gently down; feel a
comfortable stretch in arms.
f. Return to knee-heel position.
g. Wobble and loosen body.

Coordinate Breathing
a. Inhale as you raise hips.
b. Exhale as you stretch forward.

13A. CALF STRETCH ON FLOOR— ALTERNATE 3X EACH LEG

Purpose
TO STRETCH ALL MUSCLES ON BACK
OF LEG.

Position
Start in round-back position on hands
and knees.

Directions
a. Tuck toes under, raise tailbone and
   stretch legs straight back.
b. Lean body weight forward and
   raise heels.

c. Lean back and press one heel down
   while other knee bends—feel stretch in
   calf.
d. Lean forward and repeat on other side.
   [When (a) through (d) have been
   mastered, try to press down both heels at
   the same time.]
e. Return to knee-heel sitting to relax
   OR
   If you find 13A uncomfortable for your
   wrists and arms, substitute 13B

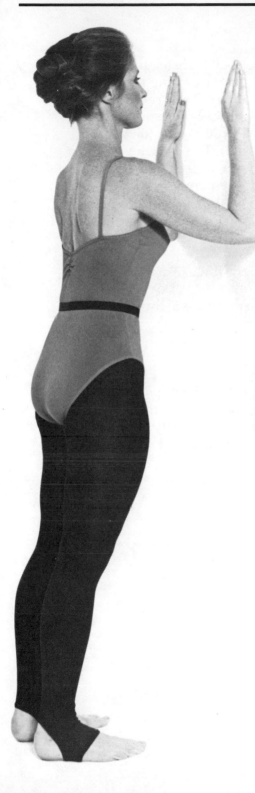

13B. STANDING CALF STRETCH— ALTERNATE 3X EACH LEG

Note
This version of the Calf Stretch puts less stress on wrists and arms.

Position
a. Place hands on wall at shoulder level.
b. Stand about two feet from wall. (You may have to adjust your distance from wall in order to feel a stretch, depending on your height.)

Directions
a. Bend elbows and lean body diagonally forward.
b. Keep belly in and body straight.
c. Keep heels on floor to feel stretch in calf muscles.
d. GOAL: to touch bent elbows and forehead to wall WITHOUT ARCHING BACK.

Standing Exercises

Standing exercises are particularly valuable because they transfer to your standing position what you've learned in basic floor exercises. The first three exercises that follow are done with legs spread wide apart. They require your constant awareness of your alignment. It is important to work through each exercise slowly and smoothly. Don't let momentum do your work for you. Don't swing an arm up to raise yourself (that's cheating!). The muscles on your trunk must do the job to develop the tone you want for a sleeker, trimmer you. Focus throughout on the movements you are making. Remember that muscles move bones, and it's the muscles you want to tone.

Before you begin, come to the mirror, and let's go over the checkpoints:

1. Ankle, hip, shoulder, ear ALL in a straight line.
2. Weight forward toward balls of feet.
3. Belly lightly tucked in; chest always farther forward than belly.
4. Center of rib cage directly over center of pelvis.
5. Back of head in line with upper back.

To accomplish steps 3 and 4 of the alignment, NEVER lean back or let chest hang behind you. Tight abdominal muscles hold the correct alignment in pelvis and chest if you are aware of standing straight. It is equally important NEVER to poke head forward—that shortens the trapezius muscle and hunches your shoulders.

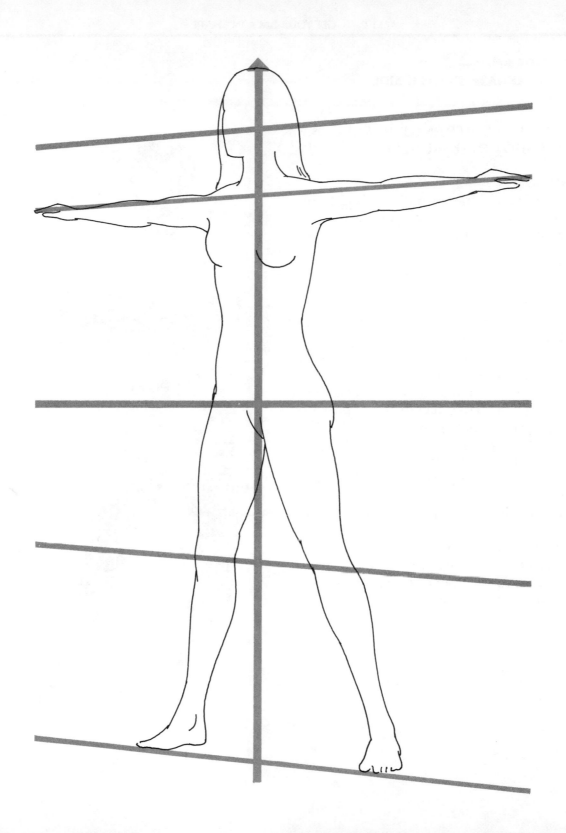

14. SIDE BEND— ALTERNATE 5X EACH SIDE

Purpose
TO FIRM AND STRENGTHEN LEG, BACK AND ABDOMINAL MUSCLES.

Position
a. Align yourself externally and pull up through the center of your body.
b. Squeeze waist in.

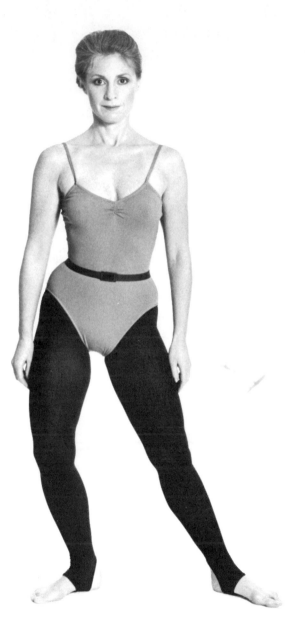

Directions
a. Tense inner thighs toward center line of body.
b. Hold tension in legs as you bend right knee AGAINST STRONG RESISTANCE.
c. Raise right arm overhead and stretch body over to left; feel diagonal pull along right side; reach chest and arm diagonally.
d. While reaching, stretch back of neck and drop shoulders down—space between ear and shoulder.
e. Return to center: pull up from balls of feet; tense inner thighs; straighten legs; press belly in; lift ribs; let back of neck stretch and lift you up.
f. Center yourself: check alignment.
g. Repeat to other side.

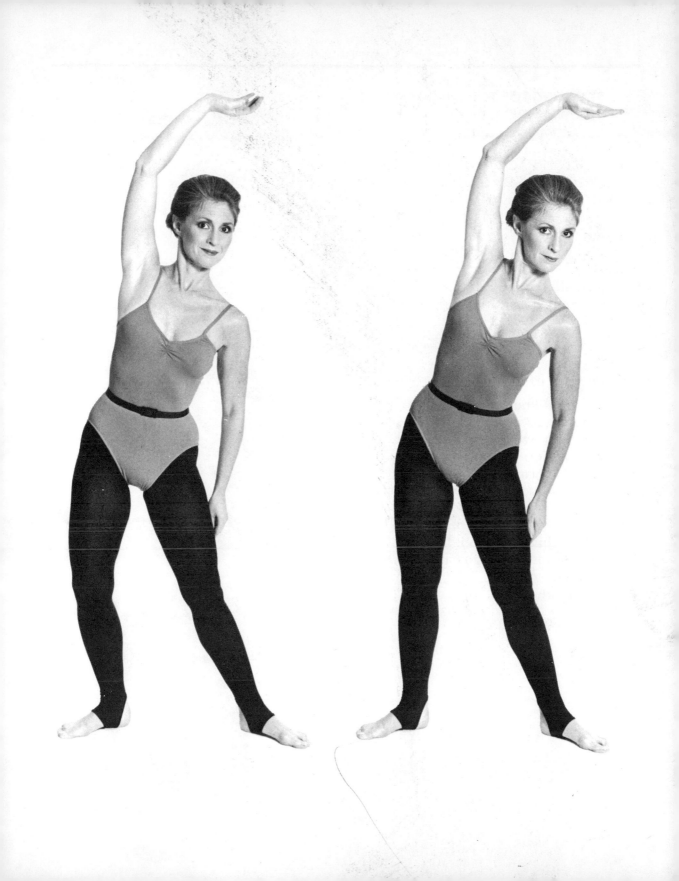

15. STANDING TOE TOUCH—ALTERNATE 5X EACH SIDE

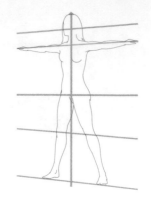

Purpose
TO STRETCH BACK AND LEG MUSCLES; RELAXATION AND FLEXIBILITY; TIGHT ABDOMINALS.

Position
a. Stand with legs wide apart, arms at sides.
b. Check alignment.
c. Squeeze belly in tightly.

Directions
a. Force right knee open (against resistance, as in No. 14).
b. Drop chest over right knee; pull head and shoulders down.
c. Reach left arm over toward bent right knee and touch leg where comfortable (knee, shin or ankle).
d. To lift: squeeze belly in; push off balls of feet and shift body weight back to center line; tense inner thighs and pull up to standing.
e. Repeat, other side.

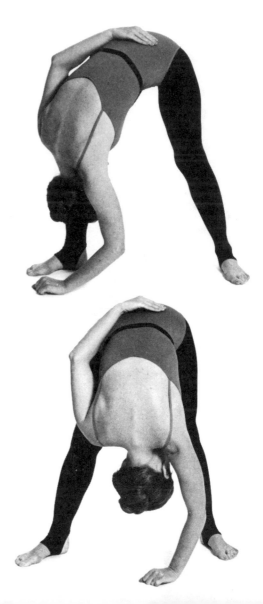

16. DANGLE-OVER HIP STRETCH—ONCE

Purpose
TO STRETCH BACK AND LEG MUSCLES;
TO INCREASE FLEXIBILITY.

Position
a. Stand with legs wide apart, arms at sides.
b. Check alignment.

Directions
a. Drop head and shoulders down to floor; press chest toward thighs; keep knees comfortably bent.
b. Slide legs wider apart, arms dangling down.
c. Stretch hips side to side, eight times, lifting tailbone on each stretch.
d. Soften knees and curl up, squeezing belly in *very hard*.
e. Inhale, exhale, and drop to floor again, to do the next exercise.

17. SQUAT-TO-STAND—ONCE

Purpose
TO STRETCH BACK AND LEG MUSCLES;
TO INCREASE FLEXIBILITY AND
RELAXATION.

Position
a. Head and shoulders dropped down to
floor, legs hip-width apart.
b. Arms dangling down.

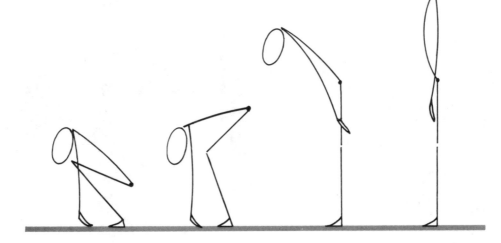

Directions
a. Bend knees to squat position,
TAILBONE HIGHER THAN HEAD.
b. Weight forward toward balls of feet, as
you
c. Bend knees and bounce rhythmically.
d. From time to time raise tailbone higher
to increase stretch.
e. Soften knees and curl up slowly,
squeezing belly in very hard.

18. SHOULDER CIRCLES AND FLINGS— EACH 8X SLOWLY

Purpose
TO LENGTHEN PECTORAL MUSCLES—
to tighten rhomboid muscles (which hold
shoulder blades and spine).

Position
a. Sit cross-legged on floor.
b. Stomach tucked in.
c. Chest in front of stomach; weight
   forward.
d. Back of neck straight, chin level; back of
   head in line with upper back.
e. Shoulders relaxed and down—nice big
   open space between ear and shoulder.

Directions
CIRCLES
a. Bend arms; place fingertips on
   shoulders.
b. Slowly make backward circles (check
   Level 1, No. 12, steps 1 to 7, to be sure
   circles are perfect).

FLINGS
a. Stretch arms horizontally out to sides.
b. Palms up to ceiling, thumbs pointing
   back.
c. Circle shoulder blades as in Bent-Arm
   Circles.

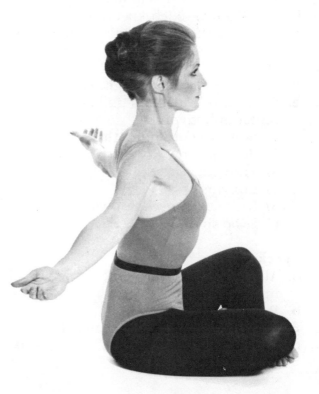

19. SITTING RELAXATION

Purpose
TO KEEP SPINE FLEXIBLE—to loosen back muscles and tighten abdominals.

Position
a. Sit cross-legged—NEVER SLUMP BACK INTO BUTTOCKS; always reach forward from under tailbone; arms loosely at sides.
b. Use pillow under back half of buttocks if muscles are too stiff to sit forward.
c. Substitute sitting in a chair if cross-legged sitting is uncomfortable.

Directions
BODY ROLL—2 or 3X in each direction
a. In a loose and flexible manner, lean shoulders and ribs to left.
b. Circle down to left knee, and
c. Continue through center, keeping chest and head as low to floor as comfortable, and
d. Continue through to right knee.
e. Squeeze in waist and pull up through center of body to lift.
 1) Squeeze both inner thighs.
 2) Pull up through center of pelvis.
 3) Through center of chest.
 4) Lift ribs.
 5) Let back of neck pull you up.
 6) Drop shoulders.

Check
a. Alignment: see that center of pelvis is in line with chest and with head.
b. Belly tight, back loose.
c. Chest more prominent than belly.
d. Sit forward on "sit bones"—don't sink back.

HEAD ROLL—2 or 3X in each direction
a. Bend left ear to shoulder and circle head down.
b. Rest chin on chest and feel stretch in cervical spine.
c. Continue circle and bend right ear to shoulder.
d. Finish circle by rolling head all the way back.
e. Keep shoulders quiet and down throughout; keep body weight forward.

Coordinate Breathing
For both Body and Head Rolls.
a. Inhale as you start to roll.
b. Exhale as you continue Head Roll.
c. Exhale as you circle down to floor for Body Roll; inhale to help you lift up.

SIDE BENDS—Alternate 3X each side
a. Sit cross-legged and check alignment (both hips MUST stay down).
b. Stretch right arm up overhead; turn palm to face ceiling.
c. Bend body sideways to left—only as far as hips stay down; feel stretch in waist.
d. Squeeze belly in and pull up through center of body to lift you up—DO NOT USE ARM TO LIFT BODY! Let back of neck pull you up.
e. When you are up, separate space between ear and shoulder: 1) stretch back of neck as long as possible; 2) drop shoulders down as low as possible.
f. Repeat, other side.

20. ARM EXERCISES

Note
Only do this series after your pectoral
(chest) muscles are sufficiently stretched:
you must be able to sit straight with
shoulders pointing to ceiling, NOT hunched
or rounded forward.

Purpose
TO FIRM UPPER AND LOWER ARMS
(deltoids, biceps and triceps).

Position
a. Sit cross-legged on floor.
b. Stomach tucked in.
c. Chest in front of stomach; weight
forward.
d. Back of neck straight; back of head in
line with upper back; chin level.
e. Shoulders relaxed and down—a nice big
open space between ear and shoulder.

Directions
a. Stretch arms sideways; drop shoulders.
b. Flex hands and raise them slightly
higher than shoulders.
c. Press shoulder blades together as you
pulse wrists farther and farther away to
the sides and slightly back (five times).
d. Turn palms down, circle thumbs under
and back until palms face ceiling
"backwards."
e. Repeat same stretching and pulsing
motions as (c) above.
f. Check position: shoulders point to
ceiling; hands slightly higher than
shoulders; shoulders DOWN; neck long
and stretched.
g. RELAXATION:
1) Arms loosely at sides.
2) Stretch from under buttocks.
3) Press in belly, drop head and
shoulders toward floor and stretch
back muscles.

21. RELAXATION AND ORGANIZATION— 3X EACH

Position

Lie on back, knees bent; feet on floor.

Directions

From Exercise 3, Level 3, select assorted breathing, wobbling. LET GO all of the tension in your body.

22. LIGHTS OUT

Purpose

To LET GO of all your muscles.

Position

a. Lie on back, knees bent; feet on floor hip-width apart.

Directions

a. Flop knees in gently; let them rest on each other.
b. Cross arms over chest and gently hug shoulders.
c. Raise crossed arms to cover eyes.
d. Be aware of checkpoints: keep belly tucked in gently; back of neck resting straight on floor.
e. Rest quietly: let arms and legs rest on each other; *let go* of muscles all over body; let weight of body sink down into floor.
f. Breathe normally and let a feeling of relaxation wash over you; let go of your awareness.

IX

Rounding Out the Picture: Stamina and Eating Well

The exercises in this book are designed for relaxation, tone and strength, for a general feeling of well-being. Exercises for stamina are also valuable and pleasurable. The great popularity of aerobics nowadays reflects how much we all want to move and be fit. Aerobic exercises are those that use a lot of energy and oxygen. They must be done a minimum of three times per week, twenty minutes each time, in order to be of cardiovascular benefit. Remember, your heart is a muscle, and, like all muscles, it will work more efficiently with exercise. The breathing which is part of the Back in Shape exercises will increase your cardiovascular capacity. But you may want to start a more vigorous calorie-burning regimen in addition. If so, it's extremely important to start moderately.

If you have back pain, many doctors recommend swimming as the safest aerobic exercise. Do you want to run? Make sure that you're NOT in pain. And if running CAUSES you pain, stop immediately! Running can be exhilarating fun; but it can also be injurious because of the constant pounding. Always take extra care of your body if you run. The Standing Exercises in Level III are excellent stretches for pre-run warm-ups and post-run relaxation. Begin by *walking* at a determined clip. Do it three or four times per week. If you have no pain, advance to ten- to fifteen-minute walk-runs to build stamina gradually. When that feels easy, advance to twenty minutes. Gradually run longer and walk less. The best rule for running, as for all strenuous activities, is: if it doesn't hurt, do it. Racewalking is a satisfying alternative to running. This is an energetic style of walking in which you establish a very brisk pace with long strides as your arms pump rhythmically in opposition to your legs. Whether you walk or skip rope, bike, swim or jog, the key is to choose an activity you

ENJOY, one which you believe in and from which you can see results. These are the ingredients of successful discipline; and only by adding some discipline to your life can you expect to see and feel your body change.

You may be itching to phone me up and protest, "But Marge, shouldn't I put off exercise until I've lost my extra weight . . . someday . . . ?" The answer, dear friend—I know you've guessed it—is absolutely NOT. Fat does NOT turn into muscle from exercise. Fat cells are fat cells. Muscles are made of muscle tissue. When my students ask me how to get rid of fat bellies, fat thighs, fat anything, I have a simple answer: exercise, eat better and eat less. Otherwise you're likely to *wear* what you eat. To get rid of bumpy patches on hips, thighs, tummy, and bottom, moderate eating is vital. Add that to regular exercise and you're sure to see beautiful results.

In addition, drinking several glasses of water through the day has been proved to keep weight down. Our bodies use 12 six-ounce glasses of water daily. Some of what we use comes with the food we eat. The rest we must supply ourselves to keep the proper chemical balance in our bodies and to help eliminate wastes and toxins.

A little rudimentary knowledge of nutrition goes a long way toward weight control. For instance, taking all the carbohydrates from your diet is NOT the way to lose weight. It's the fats that fatten. Your body is constructed to break down carbohydrates and to use them immediately as nutrients for energy. Both professional athletes and dedicated amateurs are now finding out the benefits of carbohydrates for energy and nutrition. Bear in mind that by carbohydrates I mean whole grain breads and fruits, not devil's food cake with butter cream frosting! As an example, take my thin and fit runner friend, who dined with me on spaghetti hero sandwiches the night before she finished fifty-fifth out of thousands among women in the New York Marathon.

In addition to the carbohydrates, proteins, vitamins and minerals you know are essential to a healthy body, please make special note of calcium.

Adults as well as growing children need adequate amounts of this essential mineral in their diets. It combines with other minerals to build and maintain strong bones and teeth and is important also for nerve and muscle regulation. When calcium is in short supply in the diet, the bones may become weak and brittle. (This is particularly true for women over forty.) A simple solution is to make sure there is a good, constant supply of calcium in your diet. Milk, yogurt and cottage cheese, and sardines and salmon *with* the bones are foods rich in calcium. Calcium-rich foods are vital to our having strong bones. They have even been demonstrated to relieve the recurrent muscle cramps some people suffer. Clearly, then, we all need to combine care for our inner with care for our outer selves. A balanced diet is as essential to our fitness as is muscle tone and contributes to the maintenance of both.

X

One Last Word

To sum up, it seems clear that we all need balance in our lives. Balanced eating, exercise, rest, work and play. We need to set up some rules and remember that they can be broken. We need discipline, and when we slip out of it, we *don't* need to feel guilty. We need flexibility of mind and body. All of us have some of this precious commodity; and we all probably would like more than we have.

Grow accustomed to working for balance in your life. Get used to pressing in your belly as you walk down the street. As you do, imagine your back spreading out to loosen tight muscles so they don't press on nerves. *Visualizing* relaxed muscles actually helps relax them. Stretch your head erect—it will remind you to feel proud of yourself. Let gravity pull your shoulders down. Throughout each day remember to release and *let go* of tension. Make this release an activity on its own.

The bonus, the added reward for your efforts, will come in extended vitality. What you master now will keep you suppler and stronger as time goes by. No matter what your age, you can begin. No matter how you feel, you will improve, freer to reach out and catch the best pleasures and satisfactions life has to offer.

About the Authors

MARJORIE JAFFE and STEPHANIE COOPER met, frolicked, exercised, went to concerts and cooked together, raised children simultaneously and became the best of friends during many green and peaceful summers in the Berkshires. Their collaboration on this book grows out of a twelve-year relationship and warm admiration for each other's work. They share a keen mutual regard for the values of fitness and good health.

Trained by and assistant to Dr. Sonya Weber, who founded the Columbia Presbyterian Hospital Posture and Back Clinic, MARJORIE JAFFE was Head Instructor in Corrective Exercise and Consultant to the Back Care Program at the New York City Y.W.C.A. for ten years. In 1980 in New York City she founded her thriving studio, Back in Shape, where she teaches exercise, therapeutic strengthening and toning. In classes and as a private consultant she has cured back and neck pain sufferers for fifteen years.

STEPHANIE COOPER is a writer, pianist, cured back-pain sufferer and longtime devotee of the Back in Shape program. Her articles have appeared in national magazines, and she is currently at work on a musical biography.